Sigma Male

What It Take to Have a Sigma Male Mentality

(Unleash the Lone Wolf and Master the Sigma Grindset to Achieve Success)

Mario White

Published By **Darby Connor**

Mario White

All Rights Reserved

Sigma Male: What It Take to Have a Sigma Male Mentality (Unleash the Lone Wolf and Master the Sigma Grindset to Achieve Success)

ISBN 978-1-77485-958-2

No part of this guidebook shall be reproduced in any form without permission in writing from the publisher except in the case of brief quotations embodied in critical articles or reviews.

Legal & Disclaimer

The information contained in this ebook is not designed to replace or take the place of any form of medicine or professional medical advice. The information in this ebook has been provided for educational & entertainment purposes only.

The information contained in this book has been compiled from sources deemed reliable, and it is accurate to the best of the Author's knowledge; however, the Author cannot guarantee its accuracy and validity and cannot be held liable for any errors or omissions. Changes are periodically made to this book. You must consult your doctor or get professional medical advice before using any of the suggested remedies, techniques, or information in this book.

Upon using the information contained in this book, you agree to hold harmless the Author from and against any damages, costs, and expenses, including any legal fees potentially resulting from the application of any of the information provided by this guide. This disclaimer applies to any damages or injury caused by the use and application, whether directly or indirectly, of any advice or information presented, whether for breach of contract, tort, negligence, personal injury, criminal intent, or under any other cause of action.

You agree to accept all risks of using the information presented inside this book. You need to consult a professional medical practitioner in order to ensure you are both able and healthy enough to participate in this program.

Table Of Contents

Chapter 1: What Is An Sigma Male? _____ 1

Chapter 2: What Makes The Sigma Male Sigma Male Different? _____ 8

Chapter 3: Making An Community _____ 19

Chapter 4: The Sigma Faces Adversity __ 29

Chapter 5: Haters _____ 41

Chapter 6: Rule #1: Quit Thinking About What Other People Believe. _____ 53

Chapter 7: Rule 18: Lean From Your Mistakes _____ 110

Chapter 8: Tip 1: Nobody Is Going To Be There To Help You. _____ 142

Chapter 1: What Is An Sigma Male?

I realized long back that I wasn't similar to the men I met throughout my life. Many people believe that they are Alpha Males, or Beta Men. In self-help literature and social media or even in news media the dichotomy between Alpha and Beta is one that most people are familiar with and confident talking about. Female-oriented websites such as Jezabel as well as The Cut feature articles about this distinction, but they tend to leave out references to Sigma males.

The consensus among experts is that there are certain males who are the most powerful, the strongest, the most stubborn. These guys are more effective in business, social settings, and also with women. They are commonly known as Alphas. The men left by the men who are known as betas. They are usually shy and quiet They may get harassed by males who are Alpha as well as women. Many people prefer to divide men into these two groups. I have made this error.

There are certain aspects in the Alpha male personality that people find disgusting and, in particular the tendency for Alpha males to come across as demeaning or exploitative, rude or loud can cause Alpha males a bad rap. But what happens to those quiet, strong people who are in the business of having success in all areas of their lives without needing to constantly seek attention, or belittle and insult other people?

"What do I have to say about myself?" I wondered. "Where do I fit?"

You might be thinking the similar question. I realized that I'm not an Alpha male, despite the fact that I've been viewed as one, and even by others Alpha males. I was wondering what kind of class I was in. I'm the type of person who doesn't get worried about the presence of an person who's an Alpha. I'll let him be a sham and then chase him in order to achieve what I would like. The different between me and an Alpha male is that the Alpha male desires to stand out for his power so that he doesn't get threatened. The main difference between me and beta is that while I will not dominate without reason, I'll also not let myself be controlled. You might have realized by now that I have the traits and traits of being an Sigma male. It's a subtle grey part of the male classification and there are numerous characteristics to know the nature of an Sigma male.

Let's take a look at an illustration of how the Sigma male will be perceived by the midst of a crowd. When an Alpha male steps into the room or space, whether in an office, social gathering, or any other location where competition takes place He is conscious about the Sigma male. He notices, but he knows that he's not an enemy in the same way that another Alpha male could be. A Sigma male is at his own level, but will not be a threat unless threatened. Sometimes Alpha males give an Sigma male the opportunity of friendship, or perhaps to become part of their group however, the Sigma male will be lonely one and would rather remain in his own way.

As as a Sigma male I have found myself attracting the attention of my personal followers. I've done this in a way that is natural, as Sigmas do not tend to seek out followers or underlings. The reason people tend to follow Sigmas is because they believe that the Sigma males have something special to provide and a different approach to present it than an Alpha male. Because of my non-judgmental attitude, I'm at ease knowing that those within my circle don't want to go anywhere or are inclined for an Alpha female to follow. Should they choose to, not a issue. An Sigma male is sure that they'll return.

In addition, I've found women who are as beautiful as the Alpha male's females. My method of getting women is different than the style of Alpha males. It doesn't place decision-making power in the hands of women. In contrast to Alphas Alpha, Sigmas don't compete against other Alphas or betas. Sigmas are known for their worth and allow women to meet them. We will discuss this in a subsequent chapter.

When an Alpha male is able to realize what he's working with, he will rarely challenge the Sigma male. There's a secret code that's not spoken among the ranks and the Alpha male knows instinctively who to take on and who to avoid. He'll prefer to dominate beta males, rather than making mistakes against the volatile and risky Sigma.

In the time I attended the school, we had an unruly bully in my class who was very alpha. He would walk around to each kid in the school lunchroom and pick on them from time times. He seemed to target the majority of people but he never appear to me. I never felt threatened by him in any way and I did not make any threats towards him. There was always an inconspicuous reason about why he should not approach me in the first place. I wasn't aware of it back then however, we were sticking to the male class system and playing our roles as Alpha and Sigma prior to the time we were aware of the terms.

One day there was a child who was picked on every time the bully appeared. The kid was aware that the bully did not respond to me, so the child decided to sit with me. He sat with me for lunch every day and later became my friend. I didn't mind being next to me and I was happy the fact that he wanted to become my friend to stop the bully from him. It didn't seem to bother me.

This is among the many characteristics of Sigma males. Sigma male. He is willing to assist anyone, regardless of who is aware about it. As a result, I requested for him to assist myself in math when I was struggling. In the end, I scored an A in my class, and he was a member of my inner circle of acquaintances.

What is the primary distinction between what makes a Sigma male and an Alpha male? Sigma males aren't concerned about being the leader or being in the social ladder. Additionally to that, a Sigma male is obscure, which makes him attractive to women. Women are drawn to men that they do not know much about. This helps to create a sense of attraction. The Sigma male is interested in being social with other people but not necessarily to be considered the best in a crowd. The majority of the time it happens.

Chapter 2: What Makes The Sigma Male Sigma Male Different?

The Sigma male is determined to achieve his goals if they are essential to him. He's willing to give up the things he requires achieve satisfaction and is motivated to do it. This is the thing that makes the Sigma male distinct.

Let's look at a typical example.

Let's say that you're engaged and your employer wants you to travel overseas to work. It's a fantastic chance for your career, however, you'll need to go away for the duration of a year. The girlfriend you are traveling with won't be able to join you due to her life here. Maybe she was aware of this possibility since you first got to know each other. In reality having such promising prospects is a major reason that attracted her to you initially. At first, she spoke about the possibility as if it was a great thing. She spoke of your professional career and the huge amount of earnings you could earn during your time away, in addition to the opportunities which would be available when you returned. Then but with your leaving coming up, she begins to get angry about the possibility that you'll be working in a different place.

As the day of your departure approaches the date is nearer, she starts to fight with you, and she reveals that she's afraid that in the event that you stay for a whole year with her, you'll be done with her. Over the course of the day until to when you're leaving her constant fights over you. She even threatens end your relationship. It's becoming obvious that she's making you feel uncomfortable even though she knows that you need to leave. This type of scenario is one that men often encounter.

A male who is a beta is one who listens to his female friend and remain in order to avoid losing her. He'll do this more than take the chance to accept the overseas job. It might be shocking for you (and it certainly will surprise the male who is a beta) that in the end the decision he made will lead her to split with him, and she'll go on to leave. Why? When a woman realizes that she can control you and is aware that you value your relation more so than the other, she'll utilize that in her favor. This means that you've accepted her demands and she will begin to perceive you as less important. She'll lose respect for you in time, and eventually break up the relationship, even when she has achieved what she claimed she wants. The majority of beta men aren't aware of the things they've done. They aren't aware that by placing their female partner on the pedestal and demonstrating to her that they are more devoted to her than they do themselves.

Another method to manage this scenario is in the same way an Alpha could react. The Alpha may handle the situation by imposing. He could tell the woman that he's leaving and she should wait until he returns and be loyal to him. He may try to negotiate his way by threats or violence. He might be able to get what you want however, who knows what tensions he might generate and what harm he can cause for the relationships? Keep in mind the words of William Congreve about the woman who is scorned: "Heaven has no rage like hatred to love turned and Hell an rage like one who has been disregarded."

The Sigma male is already worked the woman out and will depart to pursue his mission because he believes it will benefit him in the end. The Sigma male isn't likely to make either of these mistakes since he's willing to let his woman go when she's not completely dedicated to his cause and mission. If his partner splits with him, he's sure that he will be able to replace her without any issue because he's sure. The Sigma male is aware of the negatives to her leaving however, he also sees positive aspects. He realizes that he'll no need to invite anyone out to dinner with or indulge in events however, he will be able to spend more money on himself. He is aware that he must be able to give up the pleasures having a romantic relationship however, he'll also be able to put aside the distractions , and will also advance his career in the process by accepting the role.

If you're a Sigma male no one else can influence his choice when he is certain that it will help him. Once an Sigma male is set on a path and sticks to it and it's difficult to get him off his course. He understands what is most important and is prepared to do whatever it takes to achieve success. As Sigma males Sigma male is a Sigma male, you do the things you are required to do, particularly if it will benefit you. The only thing the Sigma male is how he can improve himself.

The above instance is only one example of a situation that shows the true character and character of Sigma males. Sigma male. The Sigma male applies this mindset throughout his life. He has a goal , and the people around him will not hinder him from achieving that target. Additionally, he is able to be free of expectations and what that most people do. A Sigma male is able to leave any situation that hinders the ability of him to achieve what he desires. Be it an occupation, a group or even a relationship, he's not going to allow other's objectives, expectations, and goals impede his own ambitions. This is the reason why He isn't a part of the standard Alpha/beta structure. He defies these limitations. This mindset can be extremely difficult because it takes away protections from the Sigma male and increases the risk for Sigma males. Sigma male, however, the Sigma male can handle these types of challenges.

Sigma Male Traits

The very first sign that you have the Sigma male concept is that of the silent, powerful kind. Your presence is automatically heard; it is the voice of the people around you. You can speak whenever you have to and when you wish to, if you want to. The Sigma male is usually more quiet than the majority of people.

A few people aren't aware of Sigma man's behavior. When they first meet one, they doubt the presence of this man. As I was starting my new job in the United States (sound familiar?) I was asked by a woman I had just had a conversation with about the reason I was quiet. I replied that I didn't have a motive to say anything. When I need to express myself, I'll speak up. She was not familiar with men whose presence speaks for itself. She wasn't aware the fact that the typical Sigma male is only speaking when he's got something to speak about. I could tell that she was used to people who were loud and talkative. The interest she showed in me inspired her to try to know me better because of my fascination with her.

This is the second characteristic that is characteristic of Sigma males. Sigma male. While Sigma males are Sigma male is able to be an extrovert and a centre at the center of all attention, she typically likes being an introvert. Beta males can definitely be described as an introvert however they do not have the ability to change from being an introvert to an extrovert in the same way that the Sigma male can. This capability is known as being an ambivert. It implies that they are being both extrovert and an introvert. The typical Alpha male is extrovert, however they can also be an Ambivert. The different is that an Alpha male gets energy by being around other people. Being validated by others stimulates Alpha males. They are in need of attention. The Sigma male is not. Many people are able to exhaust this Sigma male. The Sigma male is more inclined to being by himself, and to stay off the radar. Even while they can attract attention and be the center of attention in in a group, they do not like this unless they benefit somehow. This is among the characteristics of their character that could cause people to mistakenly characterize Sigmas. It takes a keen eye to distinguish an Sigma from a crowd.

Sigma males design their own path through life. They realize that no one else will take care of them and they must make themselves. The Sigma male isn't content with the average; he understands that it is his responsibility to create the opportunities they want for themselves. This kind of lifestyle requires a huge amount of concentration. People who are in his life seek at distracting the Sigma male frequently. This is why he often has his accused of being unfriendly or aloof. But the Sigma maker doesn't seem to take any of that into consideration. He's happy to live his life the way he wants and let others make whatever decisions they like.

You may think this would render an Sigma male cruel and uncaring and cruel, but you'll be surprised to discover that's not the situation. The typical Sigma male is usually treated in the same way he'd like to be treated. He doesn't slander his fellow men or his female companions since he doesn't need to prove himself superior to anyone else. Since he doesn't have to constantly strive to be better than everyone else He can treat all people equally.

Another characteristic that is characteristic of one of Sigma male is their curiosity. Since they have to take charge of their own life's journey they are at peace, contemplative and interested in a variety of subjects. They realize that they must be. They aren't sure that established systems of the world are keeping their best interests in mind, which is why they study the world to help make their own choices.

Although they are talented naturally charming, charismatic, clever, curious and attractive to the other sexual partner, they often be reluctant to take on leadership roles. They're focused on their own personal journey and not others. They stay clear of those occasions since they don't want to be criticized by other people, to be held accountable in a way that is unfair or be required to live up to the expectations of people who they do not consider to be equivalents.

While there are exceptions to this However, the Sigma male typically puts their personal requirements first. They're not usually self-sacrificing, like I wasn't in my decision to refuse my opportunity to travel abroad. The majority of Sigma males are driven by their personal interests at the expense of other people's needs. This is the way they find satisfaction.

The term used to describe Sigmas is "lone Wolf." The reason for this is due to the fact that Sigmas doesn't spend all of the time trying to be competitive within various hierarchy levels. He prefers to wander around for himself, to locate refuge on his own and then select mates based on his own personal criteria. The value of a woman is based on the amount of men trying to attract her attention while Alphas are distracted by competing with women they don't even consider attractive. The Sigma is able to appreciate things that aren't in the social norms and expectations. He chooses a car for the reasons he loves what it has to offer and not simply because people tell him it's a reliable car. He chooses a career that is interesting to him, reads books that he believes matter to him and spends time with people that he considers to be intrinsically important.

A rebellious Sigma male is able to truly achieve freedom by refusing to accept the values imposed by the masses. He can be in the present and create his own personal style to be who he is, and design the future is his dream.

Chapter 3: Making An Community

You'll soon begin to understand the characteristics of you think a Sigma male looks like. Sigma males are a bit different. Sigma man is the single individual who conducts his business, and doesn't let people get in the way. You might think that this lifestyle could be isolated however Sigma males are able to have their own way of creating an entire community.

The primary and most significant benefit that the Sigma male can enjoy in forming an environment is that people who surround them admire him. While he isn't looking to be noticed by others He is highly regarded in a way that is higher than other males. When he interacts with other people, they sense his presence. People instantly think of him as one they can count on. After they've met him, they realize the Sigma male is someone that they can trust, and it is worth taking the time to get to know. Being an Sigma male isn't only about dating. It's about being a positive participant in all aspects in his daily life.

A Sigma male shows charisma and leadership when others are close to him. This is the reason Sigma males are thought to be emotional skilled. They are able to manage, express, and understand their emotions. Additionally, they are capable of handling interpersonal interactions with sensitivity and discretion. Because of their emotional intelligence, they are aware of the people who are worthy of his time. If he is of the opinion that you aren't the kind that he would like to remain in contact with and will avoid contact from people who don't bring his value. It's not in the sense that the Sigma male attempts to be clear about what he does however the Sigma male doesn't want to be in contact with those who don't agree with his ideals. People who are negative or even a burden can tell from the Sigma male's behavior that he does not want to be irritated by them, or would prefer the same type of person around him.

This is the reason this is why the Sigma male has his small circle. Certain members of his family are separated from him in the event that he believes they do not bring something to his daily life. This isn't because he hates the large family, but a Sigma male isn't interested in entertaining people who are not good for him. Even family members who are close to him could cause headaches or cause serious problems in his daily life. A major and crucial aspects of becoming an Sigma male is to manage the negative effects of these harmful people without causing major divisions. He isn't looking to destroy your positive energies.

The ability to create an inner circle is a talent by itself. If it seems that you know a lot of people, be assured that the majority of people he meets are just acquaintances. They're not members of the immediate vicinity who have a close relationship with him. Close friends might know about him and could benefit from his knowledge in some way in terms of experience, knowledge or knowledge. The reason why he keeps them around him is due to the fact that the Sigma male is a person who enjoys having a conversations with others on the same level. You must know something that he doesn't know, so they'll want to keep you in his company. It is a fact that a Sigma male needs to be at ease off of you to get him to be drawn to hanging around with you. He won't befriend anyone merely because they're famous or have lots of money. He believes that the greatest people people who are loyal and reliable, whom he is able to connect.

Furthermore to that, a Sigma male can complete tasks without waiting around for someone else or trying to impress others. The people who aren't worth his time can't join his club.

The Sigma male is usually an introvert. An introverted Sigma male enjoys being alone and isn't doing it because of his social anxieties or simply because he isn't a fan of people However, he's confident and certain of his own self. He doesn't require constantly entertained by other people.

The Sigma male is comfortable in a group of people, however, he doesn't need them to prove his worth. He doesn't feel unsecure that he has to always be reassured by his friends or be viewed by other people as well-known. He is happy within himself, and is as capable of having fun and finding peace in his own space as he is with other people.

It is this tendency paradoxically, that draws individuals to his. For certain people there's nothing more attractive than being unnoticed. When you are a Sigma male is unassuming and independent There are plenty of people who are intrigued and would like to discover the unrestricted lonely. It's a lot much more challenging to achieve since a lot of people have their eyes on what they like and would like to have, but the real Sigma male adheres to the "if you like it give it up" way of thinking. He is aware that if he's designed to have a relationship or a job or even a partner the opportunity will eventually come to him.

The thirst for Knowledge

You've seen the guy who appears to know how to play almost every game played at a party or has a tiny amount of experience in fixing things and also cultivating plants in the garden? There are some guys around the world who seem to have a good grasp on the subject of almost all. When you come across these people, you're likely to switch topics from subject and the person doesn't miss a beat. They'll discuss jazz music from the 1940s as well as the international relations scene, traveling advice, or even the roster of your team of choice. Have you ever encountered such a person? If yes, then you might have met the Sigma male.

The most essential and fundamental characteristics for one of the most important characteristics that characterizes the Sigma man is the passion and desire to learn new things. The desire to learn makes him a master of all trades. While he might not have all the knowledge but he has the desire to know the most is possible and learn more about the subject that has always stimulated his curiosity.

A Sigma male is interested in doing research and learning about subjects they are fascinated by. He understands that he needs to learn to succeed and enhance himself. The process of learning helps him communicate and connect with people who are more different than his own. For instance the Sigma male could attend any high-end social gathering or party with intelligent businesspeople who might have been to Ivy League schools and he can engage in deep discussions about current political developments and the nature of being as well as big philosophical concepts. This is due to his knowledge of nearly everything. After working his brain among the elite Ivy Leaguers and academies, he is able to join in the typical hangouts and gatherings that allow groups to discuss everything from pop culture to celebrity and sports.

A Sigma male can communicate with a variety of individuals and have a great time. He will be able to enjoy himself regardless of regardless of what topic that he is able to discuss or that he simply listens. The Sigma male can play a game whenever the player wants to and, If he's motivated to play, he'll. A Sigma male doesn't play just to be a part of the crowd and he is already a part of the group simply by being there.

The most interesting aspect of The interesting thing about the Sigma males is the fact that, even while he may appear to be knowledgeable on many subjects however, he does not boast about his knowledge or show it his knowledge to others. This is another characteristic of the Sigma male's mindset. The Sigma male has a natural aversion to overtly ostentatiousness and isn't an overly confident person. It is possible to mistake him for shy, but he's in reality an introvert. Alpha males are typically an extrovert who employs his bold and bold persona to attract attention or at least to attract attention and appear domineering. The beta male is quiet. It's not because of a desire to be shy however, it is more from a position of fear. They fear being the centre of attention and be exposed to public scrutiny. They fear failing. While they appear as if they're introverted and shy similar to the Sigma male however, they're quite different. Although both the Sigma male and Alpha male seem very different but they actually are more alike than the beta male to or. Both utilize their inherent talents and tendencies to obtain what they need from social situations. As the male who is Alpha trying to keep the attention and focus of the room in order to appear important and significant while the Sigma male is quietly examining the room in order to determine what he can do to best utilize the situation to suit his own desires. This is the biggest difference between the two. The Sigma male always tries to be strategically minded. He is a good observer, makes choices and choices. He is more proactive than reactive. Thus, while the beta male is afraid to be in the spotlight in fear of failing, and the Alpha male shouts at the camera and on, the Sigma male is waiting for his moment to speak, when it is most advantageous to him. He has prepared to be ready for the moment. He has studied and read and have gained experience across every aspect of life, so when it's time to become the center of the spotlight, he's well-prepared. He will do it at his discretion.

Chapter 4: The Sigma Faces Adversity

Everyone is confronted with challenges at times. Certain people face it every day and others can avoid it for long periods of time. But, nobody will avoid it forever. Everyone is challenged in various ways. The male of Alpha might exaggerate his chest and show off when confronted. He may become aggressive and take to beating his chest. He could be threatening or claim that he is dangerous or powerful. Beta males might attempt to figure out a way to cover himself, literally or metaphorically. The beta is known for his ability to transform into the turtle, and then slipping into his shell, hope that the threat will pass. This strategy can be employed to combat adversity however, the Sigma male generally takes an entirely different strategy. The Sigma male is unique in his method to handle challenges. The primary characteristic for the Sigma male's attitude to challenges is his cool, calm and collected manner. The Sigma male remains calm when under pressure, and only responds only when he is forced to. He knows that there is the consequences should he respond to the stress of a circumstance, like being challenged by males. He'll stay clear of the situation when he is worried that you are going cause him trouble. The Sigma male doesn't like getting involved in small-scale conflicts. Whatever the situation the Sigma male is able to take the initiative to show that he's not afraid. When you Sigma male is angry it's difficult to soothe him particularly if he views that you pose a danger to people he values.

An Sigma male is extremely secure of those in his circle. He prefers to avoid situations by first providing an indication that he's not to be questioned. Most of the time the Sigma male needs to inform his adversaries that the fact that he doesn't fear him.

The hallmark of a balanced Sigma male is that he is self-controlled. This is something the Sigma is lacking in the Alpha male does not have. The Sigma can harness his energy and uses the power of foresight to anticipate outcomes and create a strategy for battle. He is not a reactive person. He is active, which means that he anticipates problems and events and plans accordingly. A male who is Alpha may sense an issue and decide that to respond.

Let's take an example. you're at the bar or at a party and a guy begins to woo the woman you're attracted to. There are a variety of options to handle this scenario. If you're male who is a beta you could withdraw and let the man in front of you most likely an Alpha take control. The male who is beta is scared of being in a confrontational situation and will look for a woman who is one that is not as attractive which is why he's less likely to get her removed. A male who is Alpha will deal with the threat of another male an entirely different manner. He could be loud and zealous, and try to draw the attention of the female to himself or provoke a confrontation with the male who is the new threat. This strategy is more likely to produce better outcomes than the method used by the beta male However, there are different avenues that remain unexplored through these two approaches.

The Sigma male's method may appear like the beta male's strategy to an untrained eye however, it's actually a highly effective approach to achieving what he desires. The Sigma male method involves waiting while watching and waiting. While the male who is intruding doing his thing while the Sigma male stays in the background and limits his efforts and is patiently waiting for Alpha to commit a mistake. Particularly at bars or at a gathering that serves alcohol, you have plenty of chances for harsh criticism. And plenty of space for the reckless Alpha male to make a mess. Therefore, the Sigma male awaits to be the Alpha male to annoy the woman, to become distracted by another woman or to defend against new enemies from his side. When the Alpha male has become sufficiently distracted, the smart Sigma male takes his time to take his target and achieves what he desires and right the sight of his foe. The woman is amazed by how smart, cool and calculated this Sigma male is, and concludes that it's the man she was meant to be with for a long time.

As you will observe as you can see Sigma male is a unique style to deal with obstacles and difficulties. He is prone to avoid conflict with his cleverness. He is a smart creature who relies on his brain first and his body later. The practice of waiting for an opponent to make a mistake the subsequent profiting from it has been around at least to Napoleon Bonaparte who said, "Never interfer with your adversary while he is trying to destroy himself." However, even Napoleon realizes that one cannot avoid fighting for a limited amount of time. At some point, even the Sigma male is forced to get involved in more or less, even a major conflict.

The Sigma male takes this occasion to make himself stand out as well. If the Sigma male is faced confronting a situation head-on, and confronts the other. He is able to adapt to the situation and knows how to deal with his own self in the event of an argument or an argument. He is able to do this without a lot of emotion which is advantageous when he must fight and is unable to stay out of a conflict. He will remain calm in the midst of conflict and will not allow his emotions to get over him. It could be that he doesn't raise your voice when confronted by coworkers or making an oath when his girlfriend attempts to make him look embarrassed publicly, or being angry when a man is trying to physically assault him and he is able to keep his cool, the Sigma male keeps his cool. The Sigma male isn't logical enough to fall into such a trap. This is beneficial to this Sigma male in a variety of ways. It allows him succeed more often in situations where conflict is escalating However, it also aids his after the battle is resolved. He doesn't hold grudges. If he loses or wins the man simply takes his own sigh and is ready to tackle the next challenge.

The Sigma male knows that being stuck in resentments and minor grievances can hinder him from reaching his goals. This is the reason he strives to avoid conflict from the beginning. When the war is over the Sigma male can move on to the next step. The Sigma male is a man who keeps things easy. It could be shocking to see the speed at which the Sigma male gets over conflicts that could cause other to harbor grudges for years however that's the thing that is what makes Sigma males distinct.

Sigmas and Relations

Sigmas have everything to do with the daily aspects of daily life. They aren't too focused on women, however Sigmas are keen on getting to know women, and even being in long-term relationships. Similar to everything else they approach it in their own manner.

Alphas usually have some kind of strategy. They are always seeking attention. They alter their voice, and manner of speaking, and occasionally turn on their acquaintances or employ intimidation to attract the woman they desire. A male who is beta is, naturally, inclined in a wait until the Alphas make their moves and go with what they can. Sigmas approach the method in meeting females and developing relationships in different ways.

The Sigma male is dependent on his distinctive traits and traits to attract women. He is distinct from Alpha and beta males. The Sigma provides a platform where women challenge his attention. One thing that people are amazed by is everybody is treated the same regardless of age or old, beautiful as well, educated, or not. He doesn't treat the most beautiful woman in the room like she's special since the fact that he doesn't offer all his power to just one woman. Once a gorgeous woman realizes she is the one who can make a difference in a given situation, she is has the ability to pick the men she would like. This is the error that Alphas tend to make. They believe that they are in control of power, but they're placing the power in those of the women they're pursuing. The Alpha is trying to find the woman he is looking for by battling with other. He believes that this will make him more powerful. He'll try and keep trying until he is successful. This is true for Alphas, to a certain extent however Sigmas are somewhat differently, even perhaps even more so.

Sigmas don't provide women with the attention they desire and the kind of attention they're so accustomed to. This could cause an anger or animosity in the majority of women, but it's not a problem. The emotion of anger isn't that unlike love. It's more beneficial for a woman to be attentive to you, rather than turning away completely. It's not always a cause for anger among women, but. In refusing to give ladies the respect they desire can trigger a sense of inquisitiveness.

If one woman is fascinated by a male, the other women be influenced and start to become equally curious. This leads to an environment of competition among women. suddenly, women don't pay focus on the fierce, aggressive Alphas, instead, they're focusing on the sly, casual and clever Sigma.

It is through this method that Sigmas are able to get the women they wish to have. Most of the time, it's exactly the woman the Alpha would fight his rival to submission to. What would they think of when they try to knock each others out even if the Sigma is heading out into the street with the girl they were fighting over?

This is the Sigma method to attract females, however the problem is what Sigmas expect from the woman they choose to marry? Sigma males are typically professional and logical. They do not think of things like soul mates or the notion of the "one sole." This kind of romantic concept is what women and beta males are likely to gravitate towards because it provides them with more power in their relationship. This means that the other person cannot quit the relationship due to the fact that there's a destiny or fate that is tying the two individuals together. When these notions are eliminated, it shifts the burden of maintaining the relationship on the individuals involved within the relationship. It means that neither should be able to relax. The Sigma male should keep providing the woman the things he previously provided - financial support and a stimulating conversation as well as an engaging lifestyle, while the woman should support the Sigma male in his pursuits.

The Sigma seeks someone with a flexible personality and helpful and is aware of how important his work is, and how she will fit in with his daily life. In the end, this is that which the Sigma male is seeking in the woman he is looking for. In a marriage that is committed to one Sigma will leave the doors open for women to choose to stay or leave as they did in the first time they met. He kept it simple and let women make their own decisions. It's this liberty for both of them which keeps the couple dedicated to their relationship. It's the belief that if they fail to keep their word to the agreement and the relationship is not going to last, it will end. This kind of relationship may be a bit unsettling or jarring for some individuals, however it's also the kind of relationship that Sigma males are likely to like to cultivate.

Chapter 5: Haters

Be cautious of his success as it could be risky. Any person who achieves any degree of success realizes that he may be a target for animosity in connection with his worldly possessions. It can result in haters. It's just normal. Males of Alpha have the same issues, but to the Sigma male the haters can be acquired in distinct ways.

One of the primary reasons that a Sigma male gets people who hate him is because the Sigma male doesn't hide his feelings when he is in a position to want something. He is the one who says what he has to say even when people around him don't agree with it. If he has a desire then he'll go out and buy it. He's so confident in the words he speaks that he frequently could hurt the feelings of others when he's not conscious of it, but not because the act is deliberate. The Sigma male may come across as harshly sincere. Although a portion of him may be offensive the emotional intelligence of his fellow man, he can pick up the slack, making him aware of what to not say and when to say it. The tendency to "ruffle people's feathers" as well as "rub people in the wrong direction," can lead to people building hatred towards the Sigma male. In a civilized society we are used to hearing what they prefer to be told. People tend to be extremely fragile and sensitive and the Sigma males eschews these expectation to be secure and sensitive to delicate sentiments.

However, these minor issues are merely superficial and on a at a surface level. There are more significant reasons that the Sigma male is a source of resentment as well as anger in others. It's due to how the Sigma male is living his life. There are some who hate the Sigma male due to the fact that he is self-sufficient and prosperous. People are inclined to dislike what they do not know. They are jealous when they observe an individual who is completely liberated, and thus the Sigma male has a lot of hatred. He is a radical change in the way society views him and exposes the lies that many people believe in. If they observe someone who can break out of the norm, then they could also If they were strong enough. Being aware that they aren't powerful enough to break out of the accepted paradigm and turn their anger hatred, anger, and resentment toward the Sigma male who has exposed the truth about their blunders. Instead of taking responsibility for to their own actions and their own mistakes rather, they target those who are a Sigma male. This is true for the beta males as well as Alpha males. Both have to adhere to the established paradigm since that's where they draw their identity however, the Sigma male is not part of this system of hierarchy. He doesn't play by the rules. He is a real rebel and therefore frightens people who are trapped by their limited knowledge of the male structure, the world as well as their personal lives.

Don't be shocked to learn that you find that a Sigma male has some haters. It is inevitable that there will be those who don't like him due to nothing else than their own fears. People who view the person as superior or different from themselves. I have encountered haters of all genders. Some I have met while others I haven't ever met. However, I've received a impression that someone isn't liking me. The Sigma male doesn't get upset by those who don't like his. He views it as compliments. He thinks it must be right for people to disliking him without cause. He accepts the negative comments of other people as a badge of respect. This motivates him to keep whatever he's doing. He'll continue to conduct his work, but he will also keep an eye on those who would like to harm him or give him a tough time or cause him to be in a difficult situation.

The difference between an Beta Male

Here's a cautionary tale. Beta males often tell themselves they're Sigmas. This is a defense mechanism that some beta males have developed to guard their fragile egos from the fact of being beta men. This could be extremely dangerous to the male who is beta as well as those around him. They might think they're in the presence somebody with a plan with a sense and the capacity to design the future they want, however in reality they're in the midst of an untruth. The beta male who claims to that he's an Alpha male Sigma is aware enough to realize that he's not an Alpha male, but isn't honest about his own self. He is unable to admit that he's beta male and is sucked to the superficial similarities that exist that exist between Sigma Beta males as well as Sigma males. He believes that he's the clever and intelligent Sigma instead of the sluggish and uncooperative beta.

Beta males will take on the name of Sigma to help getting approval and validation from other people. This is the initial warning sign, since the members of a Sigma should never ever perform this. Sigma males usually find no value in the approval of other Sigma males. They are able to take it or decide to leave it. They can only get the approval of other people when it gives them something different.

For the males in beta, (and the Alpha male too) receiving approval from other people is usually an end in it's self. For Sigma males they're always analyzing the news in an attempt to understand how they can utilize it to their advantage.

Beta males who appear to claim to be Sigma men, or lie to themselves to claim that they're Sigma males and make a huge statement about the fact the fact that they're Sigma males. It is ironic that actual Sigma males do not pay attention enough to the designation or the underlying paradigm of the male hierarchy to be able to recognize themselves as the Sigma male. They don't want to be labeled however, it generally doesn't matter to them. Beta males don't wish to be beta males and insist they're Sigma males. They usually cause Sigma males an undeserved reputation.

Beta males realize that the true Sigma is shy and doesn't have to be loud like the Alpha. The male of Beta is an introvert too, but his silence is rooted in the fear of being alone, instead of a place of education and strategic maneuvering. Beta males will say that he's silent because he's thinking or being introverted, however, in truth it is because he is scared. This is another sign that a beta man is trying to appear as the Sigma male. Sigma male.

The truth is that Beta males don't be willing to take the risks that true Sigma would. They will not break the rules set by society on them. They will not take charge of their lives. They'll continue along their course stuck in a job that they don't like and getting being married to someone they don't like and allow the world to dictate their lives to them, while insisting that they're Sigmas.

Sigma males don't even care about the term. They're too busy improving their lives and discovering the world around them to ascribe themselves to a persona or identity. Although Alpha men will go to great lengths to prove they're Alpha males and beta males will do whatever it takes to prove that they're not Beta boys, Sigmas avoid the entire debate in an authentic rebellious fashion.

The need for labels often stems from the feeling of being insecure. Sigmas have confidence, self-esteem, and self-confidence to disregard labels and think that they are not important.

He gets what he wants

The last (and possibly the most significant) Sigma trait is that Sigma identifies ways to achieve what he desires. When he spots something she wants to purchase then he will buy it. If he isn't able to afford it, he'll plan until he can afford it as he is certain he will keep it for some time. He will not purchase a cheaper version. He'll wait until he gets the one that he believes will be the best fit for the needs of his. When a Sigma male purchases something, be it an instrument or garment, or even a vehicle, his aim is to never have to purchase it for a long period of time, or even. The Sigma male will take care of his possessions.

You might be thinking what this has got to do with have to do with the Sigma male's relationships, career or even his personal life. This is the way the Sigma male approaches everything in his life. If he is in the mood for something, he'll take it to the store and purchase it. When he has what he desires then he'll take care of it and hold the item for an extended period of time possibly for the rest of his life.

This is also true for women who entice him. Being an Sigma male, he's not afraid to speak with women he thinks are attractive. He won't spend time with women that he doesn't like, with women who don't like his style or with women who don't praise his appearance. A majority of men are willing to sleep with any female so long as she's got the tits and an ass. Their sole motivation is to have sexual relations with women, no matter if they're interested in them or otherwise.

For the Sigma male, he's in a position to see the girl immediately and determine if he wants to be sexually involved with her or if she is viewed as a possible girlfriend (if you want one). Sigma males won't hang out with a woman who isn't interested in or be in a relationship just because she's liked him. As an Sigma male, he looks to a woman who is of high quality that excites him. In addition that he is seeking a lady who is able to hold lively conversation with him.

It's very difficult for an Sigma male to fall in love with a woman who he believes to be attractive or boring. If he does to meet her, he will feel uncomfortable and desires to leave the relationship as quickly as is possible.

An Sigma male's guidance comes from the Universe. the Sigma male believes that there always exists an higher power who assists him. This higher power meets the Sigma male with the needs he requires by asking. All he needs to do is glance around him. He can see the world around him. Sigma male is aware of the opportunities in the world around him. He is aware of the phrase from the Bible: "Seek and ye will discover." The Sigma male believes that the universe will always steer him to the right direction and he adores the universe as he believes there will be rewards. The universe is always able to provide options in the event that there is a problem. This is why the individual is able to adapt to his environment to make the most of his circumstances.

For instance, he does not feel anxious when is it about cash. If he's lost money due to unforeseeable circumstances or has spent more than the amount he was supposed to the money, he's confident that he'll be able to claim the amount back. In the past, God has offered opportunities that allow those who are a Sigma male to make up for what he's lost. The Sigma male is aware of the world around him and the options at his disposal. He is always able to utilize a situation for benefit himself, or identify a situation that can help him. It's up to you as the Sigma male to take advantage of the possibilities given to you.

So it Is the way an Sigma male tries to achieve what he needs. He seeks out his innermost thoughts and is open about the things that matter for him.. He takes a look around and conducts the right amount of investigation to locate the location, person or thing that is most suitable for his desires. He analyzes his resources, and determines if he has the necessary resources to obtain what he desires He goes out and obtains it. If he isn't able to have the funds and time while he thinks about strategies, and creates capital. He is ruthlessly and rationally moving ahead, step by step in order to get the things he desires. This is the thing that is what makes the Sigma male different. It is the reason he's unique.

Chapter 6: Rule #1: Quit Thinking About What Other People Believe.

Yes, I understand it. It's it's easier to say than do. The same thing that all the other people say, just get up and move on. However, we're not taking that route. We will explore the subject in depth so that I can tell you why you shouldn't. Take it as a lesson.

Let's begin from the beginning. Consider why you would like to be loved so badly. I'll give you a few possibilities: your parents weren't nice to you, you want attention as a child, you've been told by other people that you have to be liked in order to succeed. You might feel lonely and you might feel unloved You think that no one likes yourself, and so you attempt to be the person that you aren't.

Whatever your motives may be whatever it is, it doesn't matter. All it boils down to one thing and that's to stop trying to fake your persona. You might not even be aware that the fact that you are doing it. It could be that you think you're just being yourself , but people still hate you. It's very easy to blame yourself, isn't it? Since the blame lies with you, which means you could punish yourself more. You must stop doing what you're doing. Today. The blame lies with you but not in the manner you believe. The issue lies with how you've been "programmed" by other people. Because your character didn't meet the criteria it was because you were different. Being distinct isn't a great thing in our society, isn't it?

This is the way it was at the very the very least. Nowadays , being unique is the latest trendy thing. Everybody is trying to stand out. You can see them with purple hair or wear baseball caps all day long and refer to it as their'style and you'll know the concept. However, being different is a fake persona also and you're bound to aren't a fan of it. Why do you choose to do this yourself? Why would you want to try to appear like someone else?

It is not my intention to tell you to become an unrepentant douchebag and go around yelling at people for no reason. If that's your true persona, then you'll need to change the way you talk. But you have to alter the way you present yourself, not fake it. This is the entire purpose. People are able to see right through your behavior. Your body language is extremely important. It is difficult to master it. You might appear to be hard, but your face and eyes say something else. Even your hand signals could be a clue.

You know, my friend, it's probably one of the reasons why you're feeling lonely. You're desperate to be loved. You don't like fake shit people and other people don't like people who fake shit, and it's likely that you're making up the shit. You know what fake sh*t does to our minds? It is hurtful to us. It also affects our souls. Since that's not what we're. We continue to fake and faking moving and eventually, we'll break down. We then feel sad. We are lost, we feel lonely, and find ourselves feeling like we're not us any more.

Of course, we'll think that way after having faked it for so long. What do you think to find out? I've made the exact same mistakes. It was like being a goofy child who has ADHD to attract the most attention. Although it was effective however, it left me exhausted. It was a complete hammer. I'm a quiet man by nature composed and calm and not a screaming jerk. But this got me noticed and that's what I was craving so often, the approval of other people. The facade eventually came down and I was with a handful of friends with people who liked ME rather than just the fake one. You changed, yeah did you not?

The point I'm trying to convey is to quit faking who you really are. Don't change your behaviour in the hopes that other people will appreciate it. It's contingent on the circumstance however, if you go to an interview, don't dress like you're at an event. Dress according to the circumstances.

I'm talking about work, school social life, any other aspect. Be yourself. If you don't think people like the person you are Why would you be around them? Yes, you are able to alter your appearance in the event that it causes you to be unhappy. Don't try to fake it. Work hard and work towards improvement, letting it develop slowly. It's not possible to change your life over the course of a single day. Sometimes, looking at yourself in the mirror is suffices to be honest, but don't get too harsh on yourself. Find out what character flaws are that is causing you to be uneasy and make changes to that. It's for YOU, not them.

Rule 2. Go to the fitness center
Yep. Of course. You should go to the gym Yes, you've been told this many times. But , remember to remain open-minded about this. I'm not going make up stories to convince you that the gym will change your life completely and that you'll be content and get married to a beautiful woman because of your muscle. I'm not a fan at all of this fairy tale. Heck even hate it. It is a bad image of the amazing message contained in this.

Let's get started this time. You've probably been to the gym, and you might visit every now and again but you've never participated in one. It might be daunting, the very thought can be enough to force you to put down this book. But don't.

You are able to skip the next couple of paragraphs if you've already joined the gym and exercise regularly, or go through it and do what you'd like.

The gym can offer you that is vital is routine. Humans are creatures, and routine is what keeps us on our toes. I'm not able to discern from the other page how sad or sad you feel, you might be on your bed all day long, your home may be in chaotic and that's probably the reason you're stuck. There's no reason to rise. In fitness, however, you have a reason for getting up. This is the one that will help begin your recovery process.

You're probably making up excuses already in your head. There is no reason to stay because of two things: A and B. Don't. I'm convinced Give it a shot If you're looking to rid yourself of depression, or to improve your life then this is the very first thing you need to do. Include this into your daily routine the earliest you can. If you haven't joined already, sign up now and read on following that.

And I am able to see your thoughts because I've had the same experience. I was so depressed that I laid in my bed for the entire day. I didn't rise to take a bite of food. I didn't wake up to shower or take a bathroom. I even peed in my bed a few times. This is how long I was. I was sleeping in my own bathroom because the emotional trauma was too much. I lost about 50kg. When I was sleeping in my own urine I was not sure I'd go to go to the fitness center. I was unsure if I could be able to get up and tackle something as difficult as that. Then I decided to watch couple of fitness YouTubers and yes it was good to hear some motivational voices however, in reality I sat in the bed. I did nothing all day. I wanted to take my life away and was more concerned finding solutions to ending my existence than I was seeking ways to improve it. Have tried it several times. So yeah, I am with you.

The thing is This is me, writing this book and exercising every week for six hours and trying to assist you. Now that you know how deep I had to dig, you may be in a position to be open to the things I've written.

Sign up for an exercise facility. This way, you don't face the problem of not having a gym membership. Since that's also one of the biggest problems. Those damn obstacles. They will ruin your life. Therefore, face them and break them. Sign up now.

Then, why do you sign up for an exercise membership? What are the benefits? First of all, this kind of treatment is targeted at becoming a strong lone wolf which is why it's called 'sigma male'. In the end, being strong in yourself is something that you must to achieve so that you not return to this useless, unproductive condition. We don't all want that.

And the gym can do just this. It's not just about building muscle, it's primarily about building character. Discipline. This is something that many may disagree with, but do not do it too much. Do it anyway. You could hurt yourself in the beginning. You might feel exhausted. However, it reveals something. It is the most crucial aspect. It's a lot of fucking until it gets better. This is the thing that the gym can teach you. It is a way to put pressure on your body, so that it will increase your. The same principle applies to your thoughts.

Then you applied this to your own mind. You took the hits and blows, and it threw a lot of stress on you. Look at what it did to you. Today, you're studying a book about how to conquer this.

Think about it this way If you enter your first gym session and you pile 200kg on the bar , and you begin benching and squatting, you'll crush your ribs as you don't have the strength. It was not the right time to take on 200kg. Now your ribs have been broken. It's impossible to go back and train for an extended period because of this. Shit.

This is also what occurred on your brain. You consumed too much shit and you did not have the stamina to take it. That's okay. This happens even to the very best of us, truly. Before I was diagnosed with depression, I was well-liked and loved. Everything was going smoothly. However, a lot of events went wrong, and I was unable to recover. It happens.

It's important to note that the gym can build confidence and helps you stay disciplined. Two factors that help make your mind more powerful. Therefore, it is imperative that to take action. No matter how awful it is, simply get up and get moving. You're tough. You're a beast.

I suggest that you begin with the PPLPPL program. There are many available on the internet. Don't go overboard with the weights, focus upon your form first. It is crucial to discover how to push yourself to achieve something that you're scared of. Find the determination.

Once you have this knowledge when you do, you will enjoy so many advantages throughout your life. There are many things you're scared of. You might even vomit due to fear. I've seen it occur. But I have learned to keep pushing forward. The gym helped me learn this. When I first began I was always feeling like I was being looked at by people and ridiculing me. If you're feeling the same way, I'd love to remind you of Rule 1 once more. Follow the rules. If you're actively striving to improve yourself be a jerk to people who ridicule you. A few kids might be able to do this and I was a kid who was a buff I admired the newcomers. People who really desired to change and put their all into it. In the course of time, I watched them get more resilient, happier, and I was satisfied in return. Particularly, if I helped to get started.

The little things you do can aid you in the end. Don't assume that you'll feel like you're at the high-levels following your first week. It will take time. The reality that you woke up this morning to get up after showering and headed to the gym is an absolute winner and beast. It's a win for you as well and is a great feeling for me If you achieved it. You're working on your own and making yourself a better version of you, just for YOU! There is a chance that you will get more attention from males and females, but it shouldn't be your primary motivation.

Rule 3: Do not set unrealistic expectations and goals

Wait, what? Expectations and goals that are not realistic? Do you think that's a mistake? Absolutely not. It is absolutely not.

The Sigma approach and this guide is aimed to help you become the best version of yourself, so that you are able to smile again. Then why would you want to put yourself back in the same position?

It's really simple, in fact. Humans are machines, we're programmed to perform things. We are required to perform tasks in order to live. It is essential to work to make ends meet We must drink, and eat to ensure that we don't end up dying, all these things are necessary to stay busy. Imagine if there were no money and no job and no work, we'd be doing nothing for the entire day. Doing nothing is something which can cause depression.

This method is employed to ensure that you are active in whatever your objective is. If you score the A for your examination, you shouldn't feel satisfied. You'll be angry because you didn't work hard enough to achieve an A+. Only be content with your accomplishments if you achieved the highest level. Anything below that will be unsatisfactory. This may sound absurd, however there is a reason to it. When we are satisfied with the things we have and stop striving for it. Because we made it. This principle applies in the gym too. It's nice to break records and I'm content for a time when I reach a major event, but I also make sure that there's a new record to follow. Since if it isn't then I'll stop working towards it.

This is the way that humans function. We're always searching for the next dopamine surge or that next high man, we are glued to it. The pace of life is so quick and we have numerous goals and many goals and ambitions. We are looking for this and to have that, and we continue to continue to fight, but we aren't sure what to do and then we're just going to quit because it's overwhelming.

This is an opportunity to beware of. I told myself that I'd like to get to finish this book in five days, but that's extremely difficult. It is still my goal to finish the book in five days. Why? It keeps me going. It keeps you motivated. It provides me with another incentive to rise next morning, and to do the work, and it provides me with a reason to start working and not take a break. Let's say I'm not able to finish this task in five days because I made that unrealistic expectations What happens then? So I will not abandon the project. Then I'll take another day off and do the most effort I can. until it's done and the work is done because a man who is a true gentleman doesn't abandon things to be left unfinished. The real man keeps going even when things don't go as planned. There are times when you may make a mistake but there's no reason to mourn that because your goals and dreams are there.

Are you beginning to realize the importance of have these tools? If you're not able to achieve your goal, you'll be in a rush. Naturally you will be able to complete things , like a test however, you should never say to yourself, 'I wish I could have accomplished more'. Never.

Rule 4 Be social

It's it's a lot easier said than done. But I'll give how that can help you become more adept at this. I went from being a shy little girl to a lovely social person too It's just a matter of time and you have to know what you have to accomplish.

The first thing to do is must become more assured. If you adhered to rule 2 it ought to have given you an advantage. A healthy body and a solid mind will allow you to become more confident. This is the kind of confidence you desire to demonstrate to the world. Be confident in yourself, believe in your strength You're so confident of everything you do you know what to do.

General advice. If it's working for you, good! However, I'm sure it won't perform like that for many people. You can't be confident in a matter of minutes. I'd like to point to the rule 9 if you would like to read the complete tutorial on that. However, for the moment confidence is the most important thing to socializing.

But it's just the beginning. You must build confidence and trust that it will happen with time. But how do you initiate conversation? And how can you keep it flowing and engaging? There is a temptation to return to old habits, in which you pretend to be someone else. But don't. Get the thought out of your mind right away. Keep in mind that it drove people away. It's not likely to make more friends this way, and you'll not be able to be able to open doors.

What you should be is knowledgeable. There's a lot of nonsense out there that you're not aware of. The people who are interested in new information. It stimulates the brain. There is no need to worry about the news that you watched yesterday, let's face it. They claim to be concerned, but it's simply a waste of time. It doesn't get them any where. This is a common error.

The Sigma male is an example of leadership. Keep that in mind. You're trying to be an example in everything however, you must also be the leader in your life. You are the one who decides what's going to occur. The reason for this is to make sure you don't break down when things aren't going as planned. But , having a foundation with friends is crucial.

So, you should be aware. What is the reason and how. What can you learn? You can find out lots by simply looking through Wikipedia articles. Explore your interests and then try to make something from it. Explore other languages. as in rule #3, don't have unreasonable expectations you can be working on. What's the reason? People will be attracted. If you are knowledgeable and can hold their attention, it could even lead to a wonderful relationship. You don't know for certain however it's more effective than trying to get them off right from the beginning. People who are aware of their flaws generally are more liked by their peers. We're we're not suggesting you pretend to be a professional. Simply exploit your passions and make sure you set the bar high. People will notice, and be interested and begin conversations. You may be able to join in conversations if you are more knowledgeable. There will be additional tips for this.

Rule 5: Go to an excellent school and raise the bar

If you can Of course. Each school system is different. Here, you can leap into higher levels, and I'm aiming for that personally. However, you might have issues with your finances that make it possible to go to a good school. You might be in your field of work or have a degree, in which case you're able to bypass this requirement. This is mostly for teenagers and those in their 20s however it can be helpful to you, so it's your choice.

So, what makes it so important? What do you think your essay says about the person you are and the things you do? It's not even a word and is a notion that is imposed on us by the society. However, we must deal with it. One of the worst things to do is be marginalized from society. It's crucial to get your head straight. This is my opinion. The majority of our worth depends on the level of our education and, yeah, it's a pain. It's a shambles. If you don't make the money, you aren't able to offer. If you're not able to give, you're not worth the time. This is the hard and cold reality. Certain commies might befriend you because of your opinions but, let's face it that we all know that it is essential to earn an education for making your mark in the society and you want to be perceived as a valuable person. This is one of the rules I find most annoying because it aims at making you appear to be something that you're not.

It is what it is. It is our responsibility to confront it. Therefore, what I'd like that you do is to go back to school and get the most of it. It doesn't matter how difficult it may be. I'm sure it's not simple. I'm sure you'd prefer to watch a film or spend time with your people, but it's impossible to be strong if we're not aware of the things. Knowledge is power and it's not just a matter of fact.

It is my intention to make sure that I emphasize the fact that. The power of knowledge is in the mind. You can say it to yourself and you'll know the truth. It is true that wisdom has always prevailed over strength. But , wisdom must be sustained by the strength. They are in balance. This is why I require you to join the training. It is important to build the mental strength as well.

However I'm not telling you to read your history textbook inside and out. However, try to improve your abilities to the best extent you can while obtaining the best education you can achieve. It's tough at the moment, but without any direction. Without a cause. However, you are building your future. The future will be thankful to me and I for doing this today. It is important to be confident in who you are.

The more you learn the more comfortable you are. The more you learn that you know, the more people will appreciate your efforts. All is connected, and it's not supposed to be. Achieving high marks is fantastic and satisfying. It provides you with the dopamine rush you need. Make the most of it.

Rule 6: Limit or stop the consumption of alcohol

It's true... it seems like you certainly do not want to quit drinking Do you? It's good to know that reducing the amount you drink is an option. I'm not suggesting to stop drinking completely. The occasional drink is fine, it's the way we live. An occasional drink every now and then is fine. But , I'm speaking of binge drinking, or drinking too much on your own sh*t.

It could be your escape from suffering. Drinking is a way to relieve stress. However, you're torturing yourself and causing damage to the body, your temple, through this. If you train all day long, or even at least every day how can you cause harm to the one body you've got? You might think that it's too late to be concerned, however that's simply not the case. You are the body that is your only one that you own.

It's not just the body that I am worried about. It's also the mind. It's basically an "upper", providing your brain with dopamine and what is the reason? What do you think you earned to receive this boost? Did you do your best did you put your body to the test? Did you buy a cheap bottle vodka and get drunk? Stop it really.

Alcohol won't help you with your issues or issues and you are able to wish for it all you like. However, you'll feel great for a time, but then you feel like it's gone. What happens next? It's back to the place you were. You spent the entire night in a state of denial which you could have utilized to improve your self. You decided to drink to do nothing with the night.

Seriously, stop making that shit. I'm talking about it. It's fine to drink a few beers but you should stop taking alcohol as a medication or for feeling better. Alcohol and other drugs can harm your liver and body. Of course everyone does awful things from time moment, and it's okay. It is not that I'm totally clean and that I don't consume alcohol. Since I drink occasionally.

The main difference is that I don't drink alcohol to make my night more enjoyable. I don't drink just to impress people. I'd hate myself if I did this. If I am told that I should drink, then denounce their sexiness. Since they don't have the power to control my body. Keep in mind that. The other person cannot and shouldn't influence what you put into your body. I'm not talking about when someone gives you a banana, or something but when we talk about toxic substances, then hell yeah.

Think about the number of times you squandered in over the past year. Consider what number of times you went out of the bar. If it's more than zero, then you have sucked it up.

Alcohol can also affect your behaviour. Refusing to drink can build character. How many can not say no to an alcoholic drink? How many can stand up to the pressure of social interaction? Keep in mind that you are living in the sigma mentality You're a lonely individual, all you need is to be. By refusing to accept, you build your character. And it's not just for other people. I am speaking to you as well. Don't take it personally. You must be able to not say no to yourself. This is the way to build the real character.

Rule 7: Stop apologizing

Do you know anyone who will constantly apologize? Are you aware of how irritating this thing is? And I'd like to dig into this issue because I've seen this happening all the time.

So, let's get started with those who apologize to every single thing. Do you know how the word is meaningless when you apply it to every single thing? This is what you're basically doing when you say sorry for something you did not take the time to do.

It's so ridiculous. People believe that they have to apologize for every single thing they've done. It doesn't matter if the act was either small or large and it's always apologize for this and sorry for that. This is just so distasteful. What is the reason you would do this?

What is the point of apologized? In most cases did you have any influence over the circumstances, or did you simply pretend to have? We all are aware of the answer to this question. A big no.

That's the entire matter. You didn't have any control over the events that occurred weren't yours or anyone other's fault. A lot of the stuff that happens is just what happens. When you begin to apologize for events that are not in your control, you appear weak. Being weak is something you don't wish to occur.

Stop doing the same thing. Take note of how often you express your regret. If you've done something wrong yes, you need to apologize. If the problem is beyond your control you should leave it.

Rule number 8: Be kind to people as you would want to be treated.

This is an extremely important practice. You may already be aware of it and I'm guessing you're following it . If not, then begin doing it.

People will be looking at your character and judge you on how you conduct yourself and treat them. Therefore, if you treat them badly then they will be sure to treat you as well. This is how it works.

There are people who are going to treat you as a shite with no reason. It is crucial to maintain a certain level of respect for them, regardless of the actions they took. Human beings are still human and you must understand that every human being deserves to be treated with respect. Every life is worthy of respect.

Don't be a total slacker and appear super cool and trendy since you have that gym membership today. You are not aware of your personal situation. You may be in a similar situation and would like to be assisted you think? Make sure you give them respect regardless of the way they behave. Try to be more attentive and stay above their current level , and when you can, push them to the same level as you. They deserve it just as just as you are. Don't be greedy, or angered.

It is impossible to discern someone's background from their appearance or an exchange. We would like to believe that we can, and some think that they do however we can't accomplish this. It is not our job to pretend to be able to tell the difference between people.

It is not my intention that you should let them walk over you or treat you like a shite. There are boundaries that can't be crossed evidently. If someone is experiencing a bad day, or who is not in a good mood Try to be the best person in the situation. People appreciate it, and it speaks volumes about your character.

This is the main thing you should be doing. You're looking to develop the perfect character. This principle sounds simple but it's so vital, everything could be destroyed if you didn't take this step. Therefore, you should be as attentive to it as you can. There will be more advice about this in the future on For the moment, you need to keep this in your mind.

Ask yourself, has anyone acted like a liar to you? Did you know the reason? It's because they usually had an awful day or were unhappy I guess? I'm not sure if I agree with that. some people can be plain snarky, but the majority of people aren't. They're just injured or broken. Similar to you, like me. The only difference is that they express their opinions in a different manner. Whatever it might be to keep your cool, keep it with respect and love. You wouldn't want the same for yourself.

If they try to attack you, of course, defend yourself. But I'm sure you've were able to recognize that by yourself. Don't be a bully and be very clear on what you mean by "line of sight" and adhere to that rule. Self-respecting people would follow this, and we want to see you become this (again).

Rule 9 Rule 9: Be sure

Yeah. Being confident. What makes someone appear confident? What is it that makes you feel confident? There are so many questions, and it's a challenge to answer in a manner that is understandable. However, I will attempt to explain it for youin the best way I can.

There are a few important factors to consider when being confident. They are not simple, but they are essential. It is impossible to live in this way without having the confidence. So:

Point 1: Stand tall.

If you've been exercising and have been working out, this should be easily for you. Stand stall-side up and keep your spine straight, and keep your shoulders in a straight line. Puff your chest out. A chest that pops out of an oversized shirt is one of the most powerful signs of confidence. It shows that you have faith in yourself and that you're confident about your appearance. In addition, it indicates that you're not scared. You do not cower. It is a popular choice because it demonstrates an enormous amount of confidence.

Point 2 Contact with the eyes.
Very important, but difficult for certain people. It's not difficult to understand the meaning of eye contact. Maintaining it when talking to others shows confidence. The way you look at or down suggests that you're scared. It appears that way at the very minimum. Make sure to pay attention when you speak with people. Make it a habit with a partner or your mom, I don't take any notice. Learn to maintain the eye contact. Do not maintain focused eye contact throughout the conversation. That's creepy. Make it a habit to break it up every now and then. You don't want to appear like you're gazing into their eyes.

Third point: Stop fidgeting.
We all do it to an degree. You just need to figure out why you do it. If you suddenly begin shaking your leg, or if you wiggle your arms, you must be aware of it and stop that shite. You look nervous or

uneasy in the situation, whereas you're supposed to be the dominant person. You might think that people you don't care but they will. They will. It is essential to stay in a straight and steady position. You could ask a trustworthy relative or a friend to highlight your quirks. After you've discovered them, you can tackle them to improve the issues. It will help you appear less anxious and more confident.

Point 4: Talk clearly and slowly.

If you speak too fast, people appear anxious. Have you ever experienced a situation in which you were presenting a talk and then they ran through their words and ended up falling off and saying a dumb or wrong or insignificant things? This is what happens when you talk too fast due to of nervousness. It may not be as bad as in a presentation however it makes the impression that you are nervous. It's not going to give you confidence. Do a mirror interview to practice your conversation. Particularly, situations that cause you to be anxious. If you've been through this before, it will be much less difficult. Another benefit of speaking slowly is that the likelihood of you slip and saying stupid shit is extremely low. Find a good middle ground.

5. Allow silence.

Nothing is more powerful than the act of allowing silence. Many people believe that silence can ruin conversations, or that the conversation is not good. This is a complete nonsense. A great conversation does not have anything about filling silences. It's focused on the content of your conversation. silences must be permitted. Don't be awkward when there is a silence. Utilize it to organize your thoughts, or think of an alternative topic, and make use of that time to come up with fresh and improved ideas. Don't be concerned about the nuances. It's normal, and it also indicates the confidence you have in your abilities to speak. That is an excellent factor in your confidence. Your body is a big speaker, but the ability to remain silent and be able to enjoy conversation is something that only some people are able to do. When you allow silences to dominate the conversation, which can make you appear confident.

Point 6: Take big steps!

Your manner of walking is a reflection of your character. If you're afraid or nervous, you typically walk extremely slow or quickly. This is evident. Your confidence will get a major boost. Keep your posture straight, believe of your capabilities and walk as if you control the room. Do not act like an arrogant person. Just walk around without doubt or fear. Do it, and prove to them you're confident. Be yourself! You're trying to present yourself to the world . But even if people don't like your presence, you don't have to worry about it. This is what makes you unique. That's what counts. People will notice this since it shows genuine confidence. Remember that and keep practicing it.

The most important question is what is it that makes you feel confident? There is no definitive answer to give you. If you apply the strategies I have mentioned earlier and you eventually get more confident in all you do , and you'll feel more confident.

However, it's not a natural process and doesn't mean you're not able to practice it and feel good and confident once more.

What was really helpful for me was focusing on my strengths. It was also the gym. I've developed a lot of character and discipline there. I realized the things I could do. The extent to which I could expand. How committed I could become. This made me feel optimistic, knowing that any challenge I had to confront that day would be less difficult than the previous one.

It was my favorite time of the year that everything was piled over me. The challenges in my life have given me more energy and motivation to train. This made me feel as a monster that I was powerful. I knew my capabilities I was aware of my strengths and that's what gave me confidence.

There is that in yourself too. It's all you have to do is find it. There are a lot of things to try and various things. Every time you do, there is something that will make you feel confident. But I'd definitely recommend to go to the fitness class. Being heavier and more muscular will make you feel more confident.

However, as a dear friend of mine once said: "It's never about the amount of muscle you carry but the way you manage it.'

Although I do not entirely agree with him, he has some points.

Rule 10: Don't smoke.

It's true, I've have said it many times, more difficult to do than said, and this is 10 times the amount. I am aware of how difficult to give up. If you're not a smoker it, then you're able to ignore this rule since you have already met the process. If not, continue reading.

I'm not going to educate you on dangers to your health. That's not what you want to do. What I'm about to say is the same thing I told you previously that: the body's temple is yours and you must take it seriously. Also, you shouldn't be smoking cigarettes because it harms the body. I've heard it previously, clearly.

Another drawback of smoking is which is the one that bothers me the most is the cost. It's expensive. What can you do to grow as a person if you're throwing your cash away to finance an addiction? This is just a weak approach. The work isn't just about growing and becoming a better person. It's as much concerned with managing money as well as making it. And if you're going to spend it in cigarettes, something I have done as well, it's an awful waste.

Do your best to quit. Do everything you can to stop. You don't have to stop right now however, you should make plans to stop soon. Because the longer you are hooked to this drug and the more difficult it is to quit. The "Doomer" lifestyle revolves around tobacco smoking, however we're trying to break the cycle.

Rule 11: Be kind to the darkness.
Accept the darkness. It is an exercise in your courage. Have you heard this before? The meaning may not be apparent, but for

me it is about taking on ones fears, and then being brave.

That's also my intention in this policy. All of us live in the darkness, and we all have our anxieties But why do we run away from it? Your mental state is not right and you're probably thinking "Oh, everything is growing on me and I'm just going to and give up. But, no. Don't do that. It's not easy but you have to face the darknessand need to stop running from it.

Greet it. Treat it as your most trusted friend. The dark should be your friend, truly. Accept it with open arms and accept it as an integral part of your life. You will never be free of a kind of darkness. It is a fact and fighting it will cost your energy. The energy you expend should be used to work, because that already is hard enough. You're really trying to channel all your energy to be focused on positive outcomes.

It might be difficult to pinpoint what your dark is precisely. You must look in the depths of your being. While it may seem evident to you, but for others it might but it isn't. Darkness could mean anything. It could be anxiety or fear, or doubt. You can run away from it, regardless of how fast you push, you'll not be able escape it.

The act of embracing darkness can also build the character of individuals which is another major goal of the Sigma approach. Consider a moment to think about the idea.

How many people are able to face their anxieties by themselves? They would like someone to take their hand and they would like to be on the television or do some other ridiculous shitshow. They are basically trying to make an appearance out of their fears or perhaps they're not sufficient. However, you are. You must be confident in yourself, too. You're not a clown that is looking for attention, but you're determined to face your fears and beat the crap off of them. That's exactly the thing you'll accomplish.

It's going to be difficult. However, confronting your fears is something you need to take on, regardless of how difficult it may be it's part of your mentality. We're going take on that challenge.

Note down your worries and doubts. They should be ranked from low to high and determine which hinder you the most. Then, go for the largest one immediately. Accept it. Accept the dark and, as you grow as a person. Build your character. It's not easy, and is more difficult to say than do. However, you must. We must.

Once you've completed that you'll see how strong you truly are. It is important to be confident in your abilities. It also helps build confidence and is the way to connect every rule. All things are interconnected.

Rule 12: Don't be a comparison to other people.

If you're like me, you look at yourself in comparison to others. When you receive an A or B, or workout, you will always look at your performance in comparison to others. It is scientifically proven that you do this to judge ourselves. It is a great way to evaluate yourself in certain situations, like at the gym. When I see someone is lifting more than me, it irritates me. It's a boost of motivation when it happens.

However, you have to be able how to accomplish this in a healthy manner. It is not a good idea to chase the accomplishments of other people. Rule 3 says to not have unrealistic expectations. However, I must ask you to demand only the best from yourself and for yourself. Other people have no part in this and you should be aware of that.

Comparing yourself with others isn't helping you enjoy life. It doesn't matter if you're comparing yourself with someone else who is better or has less luck. Don't also elevate yourself due to the misfortunes of others. It's simply a joke and is against the ethos. You must be lifting the other person up.

When you judge yourself against someone else, you are putting yourself in a position of disdain. What's the reason? It's a bit stupid to do this. You're working your a** off, you're working and doing your best. If someone is doing better doesn't mean that you are doing less than you, unless you don't do your best. It is my assumption that you do, and that's all you have to do and that's all you need.

Let's be real for a moment here, too. Like you, you dress up in this facade as do other people. They present you with an altered version of themselves. They believe that they appear to be the most perfect version of themselves. They're faking their actions and, as I mentioned earlier it's mental torture. However, be aware that what you are seeing is most likely not real.

It's human nature to think that somebody else has a better lifestyle that we have. The saying goes that the grass always grows more green on the opposite side. It's true that you cannot compare yourself to other people such as that because you may not know their names or what they go through. Be aware that a lot of people cover up their feelings and struggle.

However What do you gain from comparing yourself with other people? You're placing yourself and your personal value at risk. At the end of the day, you'd like to live an existence that is satisfying, isn't it? This is the reason you adhere to these guidelines to make your life meaningful once more. It is to have something to get up to. Instead of comparing yourself with others and trying to take a lesson from their experiences. Examine your own values in comparison to those of others. I'm talking about who you are and what you would like to be, the kind of relationships you would like to establish, and what you would like to remember yourself. You might gain some fresh insights. But don't view it as competition, because it isn't.

If you continue to compare yourself with others, you'll be in a losing fight for the rest of your life. It's not likely to make you feel happy. It is inevitable that there will be someone in the world who's more successful, better and smarter, more muscular cool, and has more friends, and there are a myriad of fields. It is important that you're satisfied with your identity and your personal values. They should not be defined by the accomplishments or possessions of someone else.

It's quite fascinating but it can be quite entertaining! Take advantage of their abilities and you could be able to enjoy their talents. You might be surprised, and it may make you new friends If you're enjoying doing it. And who is to say, they could help you learn things that could have taken longer when you were doing it all on your own. Be sure to view the abilities of other people as something that is positive. Chances are they would like to encourage you as well. Take advantage of it, as these opportunities are often scarce.

Therefore, I'm asking you to be aware of this. You're probably doing this a lot. It's true that he is lifting more weight, and there are more of his friends. You're doing yourself an injustice. In reality, you do not gain anything from this. Try to keep that in mind. Try to think of the situation in a positive light. You could ask the guy who lifts more, what they did to lift more weight. Also, be thankful with the person since they are working to improve their own. You can utilize that negative energy for many other positive things. It's not easy to alter that thought process within your mind But you can make it happen.

Rule 13 Use your anger as an instrument

Alright. What's the reason? What's it? What causes you to be angry? Does it come from a spark in your soul? Are you enraged with the universe? What's happened?

I'm sure a majority of us are very angry. Very angry. We feel abandoned and not understood. It was a struggle for me for years. I always wanted to smash things. However, it made me think about. I'm pouring all my energy into this anger. I am feeling sad, angry You know the drill. It's not solving anything.

It is not a good idea to be angry all day long. If you're suffering from anger, you should seek therapy. It's going to end your life in the near future. If you're like me, or just mad about the state of our world, and the way the world is going keep reading.

Anger can be a positive thing. It is a sign that you aren't satisfied with your current situation and that you would like to change things. This is the first step in this crap. The whole thing won't work without anger. Make sure to irritate yourself before you get started with all this.

Anger can be a source of motivation. When I feel down I enjoy it. It's not a good thing as a couple of months ago, I would be lying in bed, feeling bad about myself. However, I have learned to put your anger around the motive of changing. I can work twice as fast at the gym when I'm angered. If I let that anger out, it inspires me to become more effective. To do better. Never fall as deeply as I did again.

Another advantage of anger, which is usually not considered because it shows your weaknesses in such a clear manner that it is impossible to overlook them. What is it that makes you feel mad? Think about it, and you'll probably think of a few items. You can make changes to those issues. You can alter these issues. You control your emotions and the ability to avoid becoming very angry about small issues. Because you resolved your issues instead of dismissing them.

It's also possible to make use of anger as a method to move. Yes, it's sort of like the concept of motivation for gym but it's far more than it is. In anger, there is a need for action, so be aware of it and then go. Do what you've always wanted to do. Don't let anger rule you. Beat it. Sometimes, anger can be a beacon on your way that guides you. Make use of it as a personal weapon.

It's also good to let loose hidden emotions. Everyone has their own personal issues that are buried there, things we're not ready to face. When we aren't able to anymore, and we must be angry. This isn't something to be worried about, perse. Human emotions are natural and normal. You just need to learn to control your anger and pinpoint those things that cause you to become angry. This will make your life much easier.

I would like you to hold a little of that anger within you, even after having discovered how to handle your emotions. It is anger that drives this mentality and it's the main weapon. You must have it. In a healthy way. Don't be fooled by the fact that you did it.

Rule 14: You're enough

I first thought whether I should add these tips to the list, but I decided to stay clear of it. This is the core aspect of the mind at the very least it's not something I would like for you to try. I want you to confidence in yourself once again. You've been doubting and blameing yourself for so long You may even have begun to hate yourself. People who are depressed tend to hate themselves, so I'm guessing that you too.

However, you are more than enough. It doesn't matter what you are or what you've done. Everyday is a brand new chance to improve things. Everyone has have made errors in the past, and we all got into this negative mindset for a reason. But ask you yourself, is it truly your blame? Was it your fault? Do you really deserve this or did you not?

The answer to that question is likely to be yes, which is quite sad. However, what I found most helpful was looking at others and what I thought of their actions. Do I want to wish anyone a bad mood? Absolutely not. I'm not even talking about my greatest adversaries. Believe me when I say that I hate this guy and everything I own. However, I wouldn't have a wish like this on anyone, in any way. It's simply too cruel.

Then ask yourself: do you think this would be something you would wish on someone else? No? What is the reason you are not worthy of this? If yes, then you should return to rule 8. Everyone deserves to be happy.

Rule 15: You're the only business you require.
This is crucial. People appear stressed or needing constant attention. It can make you appear weak. It looks stupid, or looks like you're not paying attention to

something. It's either way, it's silly and you should not focus on the other people. You are the main person in this world.

We were created alone in this world. We'll end up dying alone in this universe. Sure, it's good to be around people. Being with friends, girlfriends or whatever, it's great to have friends close to you. You aren't looking to be isolated. However, and this is a big no-no don't depend on them. They won't be always there to help you always and we all want to believe that they are. We all know that's not the case.

You must learn to operate and construct things by yourself. You've already begun doing it by attending the gym, which is the first step. It's an integral aspect of your daily routine. Just accept that there will be times when you'll be all alone. It happens to everyone. It's true that they're not always enjoyable. It's true that they usually suck quite a bit. However, if things turn bad, you could be left on your own. Even if the situation is, you'll always have a plan B. Do not ignore that issue because if it occurs you'll end up getting fucked which is not something we want to occur.

It's not fun to be alone, however you can manage it. Being alone does not mean that you're alone.

When I'm alone, I think about the things that I like. Any time I am free with my family and friends, as well as gym or school is utilized by me. It's mostly for working on this book however it really assists. I'm working toward one of my goals, and this keeps me active. What should I do if I'm not completely alone? It's my path and destiny. You must be a part of that too.

It's not worth your time if you're bored. It's not that you have to continue to scream or playing throughout the day, however, you should be in a position to be occupied in order to develop. It is best to work to achieve your goals throughout the day long.

It's true that this isn't real and it's not in the same way however, once you have this mindset, it becomes effortless.

A few more things I could say to you: if you are feeling uneasy, take a media break. It's as real as it gets. It makes you feel low and lonely, so make an effort to cut that shit out. You can also think about what your ideal date is or what you'd like to do with your acquaintances. Have fun alone.

Yes, I know that it's because you're not making new friends and are still feeling alone. However, you must discover how to be happy with yourself first. If you don't, then you're lacking confidence, and the whole rules don't work.

Rule 16 Rule 16: Be kind to animals

Animals are companions. The animals are friends. We are animals.

Okay, I'm not talking about how to take care of your cat , dog or your hamster. Of course, you should. However, this is about life in all its forms. You must learn to appreciate life in all its kinds and shapes. It doesn't matter if it's a fly, cat or spider Be kind to the creature.

And this isn't to support a weird spiritual or vegan lifestyle. Not at all. It's possible that you don't see the significance of it right now but in time, you will.

Respecting the life of others starts with you. The first thing that you've ever observed. As a child, you were surrounded by various animals that were alive. Did you ever get hurt without warning? Perhaps they were playing? Did you ever get attacked without any motive by them?

I'm going to refuse this. That is how we're trying to live too. We have our own goals and so do the people. They are trying to be able to live, but we are more about the bigger picture. However, we do not harm or attack things without a reason. We just focus on our objective and If something gets blocking our path we take it down. However, we all focus on one thing, and that's our main aim. We have a reason to fight.

We're actually not all any distinct from the other species. Respect them as you would treat any human. Once you've learned to respect the lives of the smallest of people you will realize how vast yours truly is and the enormous potential you hold.

But how do you know if you have potential even when you only destroy and kill? Are the fly or spider harming you? It could be that it is triggering something inside you, the need to take it out?

I enjoy comparing them with the challenges that we have to overcome. Instead of addressing them, we degrade them. By doing this, there is no room for development. Then we kill it and then eggs start to pop out and create more obstacles in the end. In my attempt to convey is that all life's worth is equally worthwhile.

It is important to treat the situation as such. Since at the end of it all, we're all made by something and that something has given us this life. It's not up to us to determine what kind of life is more valuable. It is possible that pets and cats can make wonderful companions too. If you show them respect, they will treat your feelings as well and show affection. And why? Simply because you have gave them respect. That's how your mind should function too. Be able to survive on your instincts. You might even pick up a few lessons from their experiences. They've survived for thousands of years, and there's a reason their instincts brought them to this place. Don't be the next dog or cat Please.

When it comes to life or death you ought to take it down it's a given. However, you don't want to be killed or injured in the name of nothing, would you? Therefore, don't do it to anyone or anything else. Rule 8 is to treat people the way you would like to be treated.

Rule 17: Be aware of your own body
This rule will be fairly straightforward however, it isn't.
Essential hygiene must be maintained. Additionally, it will boost your self-confidence. Brush your teeth at least at least twice a day and shower each day, and don't allow harmful substances into your body without reason. For whatever reason, don't take it on.

If you're working out, you're performing more exercise than an average person is doing to improve their health. That's great in all honesty. You're far superior to them. You must keep working at it.

Be sure that your diet is healthy and correct. In this section, I will provide more about exercising and eating right, but to follow this rule of thumb be sure that you are getting enough calories. Don't go too high, and don't go too low. Try to maintain your weight and keep in good shape.

The grind is hard. It's a battle that you have to fight every day. You will require every ounce of energy you can find to get through the initial stages. You'll need food to fuel this. Also, ensure that you're not starving yourself. You're not.

Always be prepared for anything. Take gum to keep your breath fresh. Visit your dentist frequently. If you're in discomfort, but don't chew through it. We want you to be in top health and you cannot be this if you're sick or injured.

It can also do greatly in building your confidence when your body is in good health. A healthy body means an ideal state of mind It's all interconnected. You'll feel happier in yourself and others are likely to notice you and it's an all-win situation.

Do not expect spectacular results right from the start. It could be weeks or months. It's fine. It's a process, and so is the whole approach. Your body requires time to adjust and you shouldn't be rushing it or be stressed even if you're not an Greek God in the midst of a day.

A healthy lifestyle gives you more energy. You're more rested, and you feel more energetic. A healthy rhythm simply implies that you are more energetic. Plus, more energy means you have more energy that you can use towards your goals and dreams.

Do you realize that feelings get more intense when you're feeling bad? It's likely that you do since you've felt like that for several months. Being able to take good care of yourself can aid in this. In the event that your body's in good health and is in good shape you'll be content and you'll feel better.

A healthy body can also help reduce mental stress, whether you believe you me. That's one more reason you need to take good care of yourself. If you can manage your mental stress better you'll feel more relaxed. Simple math.

Last but not least you will be healthier! This might not be the most appealing news to hear now However, once you've adjusted to the new way of thinking and lifestyle, it's. If we live longer, and are healthier are the more difficult it is to endure. This brings us further towards our goal and ensures that we can live a happy life. It will be evident in just a few months or weeks. It's possible to live a beautiful life. However, I'm really begging me to care for myself today.

Chapter 7: Rule 18: Lean From Your Mistakes

It is difficult for us to accept that we do make mistakes. Particularly in this way since we are trying to make sure that we do everything correctly and do the best job that we can, and you might believe that mistakes are not a part of this. It could be logical however, errors constitute the majority of the mindset.

Everybody makes mistakes. There are those who make minor mistakes and others make big ones aren't important. The concept behind mistakes is to learn from mistakes. There is no way to be perfect at everything even though you are so obsessed with it, you'll make mistakes throughout the process. Your path is bound to be filled with errors. While that might seem, you don't need to worryabout it, since the good news isthat we have the ability to take our lessons from mistakes.

This is the tough part. If we are looking to learn from our mistakes then we have to accept that the fact that we've made mistakes. This is what I have learned from personal experience. how difficult that is especially in our circumstance. We're already feeling guilty and feel guilty for our mistakes of the past.

The past, however, is just that, the past. Let the past go. You're a brand new person. This new person is bound to make mistakes and admit to the consequences.

That's one of the steps. Acceptance. Don't try to hide the error. Accept that you've committed mistakes. Recognize it and apologize to the people you've hurt or harmed. Also, offer them a genuine apology.

The way you think about your mistakes is how you reflect on them. You must reframe your mistake. Don't get all negative about it. It's wrong making mistakes. We all make mistakes and most likely you didn't have any intention of this happening. It's okay.

When you've realized your mistake and you've figured out what went wrong then you can consider what you can do in the future in order to prevent repeating the same mistake. It's as simple as this. Don't be a victim of this nonsense. It's not possible to be positive and we can't continue beating ourselves up as we need to keep going. Consider what you can learn from this error. This mistake has changed your life and made you a better individual.

Ask yourself five reasons why you made the error. It is usually possible to pinpoint what is the cause of your issue. If you're tardy to work, why? It's because you slept too long. Why? You slept late. Why? You were up late. Why? Because you were gaming? Why? Because you were bored, etc. Continue to do this until you pinpoint the problem. Then fix it.

The most crucial thing is that once you've learned from your mistakes and examined them, put them into use! It's not enough to just acknowledge it, rather you must change the way you approach it. This is the most crucial aspect. Make the change immediately and adhere to the changes. Don't make the error.

Rule 19: Be aware of who you really are.

Whatever you're like. No matter where you came from. Everyone has a past. Some are more dark than others. It does not matter. Your mindset can shape you into a completely new person, but that does not mean that you have to abandon the person you were before. Only the bad qualities or negative beliefs.

The past you is the basis of the person you are today. The previous you struggled hard to get to what you're now. And even if you're satisfied with the person you are currently, you're trying to be the most perfect version of you. And you wouldn't be able to get to this point if it weren't for the former you. Remember the person you once loved. It's still there and you need to be able to accept and respect its presence. Relish it, even.

Particularly your character and character characteristics. Your character is still there. You're trying to get better and reach your goals. It doesn't mean that you're in the process of killing yourself Absolutely not. It's just about making the old you the best version of yourself.

The person you are today do you feel satisfied with your current self? No? Work on it. When you are ready to give up, and every moment you feel you're not able to continue think about the previous you. Do it for the person you love. It's impossible to fail the previous you. It's impossible to return to the state you were in. However, you need to be aware of the person you're from and also where you come from. This person still relies on you.

Rule 20 Rule 20: Be around like-minded individuals
Read books about your goals, particularly by people who live the lifestyles you would like to live. Develop something you believe in make a mark in the world. Establish relationships with like-minded individuals with similar goals to your own. In the second, you need to train. Choose what you would like to be prior to starting lifting. Adopt a proper diet and exercise. Healthy eating is only one aspect of. Don't be intimidated by the opinions of others. Keep your routine consistent as you

increase your workouts every week. The outcomes will soon be evident and you will gain a new feeling of confidence. Consistency is the key. Finally, true love. Don't fall for social norms on dating, and feeling guilty about missing out. The quality of your relationship is more important than the quantity. Find a genuine connectioninstead of one which is based on your values in life and what you are able to offer. It is important to ensure that the relationship you have with someone inspires and helps you on your pursuit, not divert your focus from the goal. Find a partner, who is not a liability' Perhaps a Chad is probably.

What I'm trying convey here is that the presence of positive, positive persons around and having people who are supportive of you can make all the impact. It's possible that you don't have them right now. I do not have them. However, I do attempt to meet people who have similar interests. People who exercise as well, and people who enjoy writing. It's important that you surround yourself with other people who are like who. And , yes, it's difficult. It's not like it's simple to connect the dots.

The way in which 'Chad describes his life sounds like something out of an old fairy story. We all want it and if it were that simple, you'd never be reading this nonsense. But that as stupid as it might sound no matter what the guy is talking nonsense. That it's not logical and it wouldn't be able to work that way.

It is important that the person has the correct mental state. The mental state of mind. Fighting. This is what we're doing. The positive energy is, even if it's not too excessive, did bring a smile to your face. It brought you to thinking about something you'd like to accomplish, someone you would like to be, whatever you want to call it. Then I'm doing nothing but negative and party-pooping. It is time to take the negativity from your life. It's keeping you from moving forward. It's a horrible curse, and you have to remove it in the shortest time possible.

So, instead of getting annoyed with Chad look for the positives in it. The attitude of the goal-setting are the purpose we're here to serve. You must surround your self with people who have this. People who think and act in the same way. There's no need to share the same goals and goals. This is, of course, beneficial obviously but it's also a major advantage if you are able to work for the same cause however it's not required. There is still a way to support one regardless of your goals. It's all about positive thinking It's about pushing and the encouragement that we need to be able to progress, even when we are moving to the contrary direction. are able to be a helping hand to one another.

Rule 21: Make sure you practice your mindset more than you discuss it.

It's so simple to discuss it. It's so easy to refer to yourself as sigma or to refer to yourself as an individual, only and later return home to feel like a shitball because everyone thought you were a weird person. You can also pretend to tell yourself you're not. Don't do it. Stop talking.

It is possible to be talking about the idea it's totally okay. However, it's not going to help you get anywhere, and you know that pretty well. Begin putting in the work.

You're right, I'm not sure what your goal is. If you want to be a lonely one, okay, this system is a good fit. If you'd like to be recognized and feel safe it's fine the system is able to do this too. But they do have one thing they share and this is that you must put in the effort. You won't succeed if you don't want to work for that crap.

People will notice the effort you put into it. It will be evident that you are working. You'll notice the changes that have taken place in you. Your body, your physique. Also, your mental health.

I have provided everything you required and more on the right track. Take this seriously. Adapt. Be brave, conquer your doubts, simply get to work. This is all I can say to you. The strength comes from you. I am sure you have it within your and you should apply it. Don't be a fool and talk about it, go and try it.

Rule 22: Never have anxiety.

One of my most favorite shows, The Walking Dead featured a line that remains with me. The show featured a particular group of survivors that went back to their primitive condition. They were affluent and adjusted to the world in the way it was.

"In the darkness, we're completely free. We are not aware of anything, we are completely free. We do not fear anything We are liberated. We embrace out death. This is the moment to end the world. We are the final chapter of the world's'

No, I'm not saying that we live in the midst of a zombie Apocalypse. However, the "we fear nothing" phrase really made me think. It's because it's true. If we do not fear anything is that we are completely in complete freedom. When we are not afraid is that we are free to do whatever we want because no really matter how it goes. We don't have any fear. We are living for it.

That's an aspect that is crucial in this mentality. Don't act as a complete idiot and commit crimes that are unjust however, you must stop being scared of certain things. It's not easy and much more to do than it is done, but once you've managed to overcome your fear, you'll be able to achieve so much more, and achieve so many things that other people can't because they fears. They're afraid of failing and leave the work to other people. For leaders, for those who can take control of their lives and be in control. That's the type of person that we must be. How do you get rid of their fears? If you Google that shit you'll find items like "Request help from a doctor and other nonsense. It's not that there's anything wrong but that's not really the main point.

First of all, you must be honest about yourself. It's hard but you must take the initiative. Accept that you are facing this fear at the moment. And also accept that you have the ability to over it. It is important to combat that feeling However, you need to admit it's there in the first place.

Once you've completed this, determine if you have control of the situation or when it's out of your control. If it's beyond your control, don't even think about it. If you can control it then it's likely to be emotions. You're likely to be doubting your self again or you might be experiencing a similar struggle. In such a scenario it's crucial to regain control. Remind yourself of the person you are. Be aware of who you wish to be. Be brave and face your fears. They won't harm you. And if you mess up it, you'll learn from it and do it again.

Also, you must stop worrying about what you think about and your surroundings. You're working hard every day. You're in a position to conquer this obstacle. You are aware of it. You've already conquered the most difficult portion of your life so far. Now, you need to turn the fear into something positive. You are able to do it however, you must affirm to yourself that you can succeed.

Another scenario. Let's say that someone is trying to fight with you, and you are feeling threatened. We're not discussing fear of physical harm, no there is a serious concern for your physical health, for whatever reason.

It's normal to feel scared in situations like this. But , you should be prepared to fight. It doesn't matter whether you're ready to fight or not, the majority of fights revolve around who's the strongest or who throws the strongest punches. Have you seen a clip where a small-sized girl talks to a man of size in high volume? She basically subdues him using words, even though he's far more powerful. He can whip her neck as if he were a pencil, but she still resisted. What's the reason? Because she's the dominant character in the scene. The guy didn't think that was going to happen.

Take care though. Do your best to not create a situation that is worse But I'd still recommend to end the situation as soon as you can. However, if you display anxiety, you've got yourself into a trap. Therefore, you must get over that. Keep your emotion under control. If you are afraid you are letting the other person know that they are the one who is dominant in the discussion.

Standing high. Be clearly and loudly. Make use of the confidence rule. And when it comes time to fighting, remember that you are fighting them. This is the only thing to remember today. You're determined to save yourself. Take on the role of an animal.

Worst case scenario, you die. You shouldn't worry about death. It's part of life and is always lurking around the corner. It's something to be aware of also.

Rule 23: Take the path that is the most difficult

Human nature is to look to the most convenient route. Everybody will advise you to go for the easiest route since it makes life simpler. They might be right. However, they are living in different conditions and therefore, how can they know what the path we take is?

I truly believe that consistently making the most difficult choices develops character. If you're used to being difficult, to having difficulties, and even enjoy the challenges and challenges, you'll be able to endure the entire world, if you need to.

You must be strong enough. I want that you be strong enough take on the world. Since the sigma philosophy does not focus on the easy way. We're not suited for an comfortable life. We are driven by to see results. Naturally, we want to cut corners However, ask yourself: even if you did not give 100% are you satisfied with the results? Or do you feel an emptiness. What happens if it doesn't work and you don't give it the effort to do it at 100%? This is a pain. You will not want to look back and regret not having done more.

Therefore, when you're able to choose between hard or easy and you're always choosing tough. It doesn't matter how difficult or difficult it will be. It's an exercise in your strength. It's true that the first few times are bound to make you feel. I'm already able to tell you that. However, the more you practice this, the more powerful you'll get. In the end, you'll be awed by the fight. Because it's a problem. We like that, don't we?

Rule 24: Earn as much money as you can
Yeah. This goes against the entire concept of this mentality. The reality of the matter is, money can be a source of power. It should be a an integral part of your daily routine.
It's not all. But it's so damn important. It assists us in achieving our goals and goals. It is impossible to enroll in the gym without paying. It's possible to try but it's not working. Other things we are concerned about such as family, education, etc. How do you plan to buy your family members gifts that aren't based on any money? How do you plan to create something completely from scratch? It is always necessary to have funds to begin. In fact, even a university education can be expensive as hell.

The truth is that money gives the opportunity to have a better life than what you're living. Then we return to the core of what this entire mindset is all about living a more fulfilling life. Money also grants an individual financial independence. There is no limit in the things you wish to do. You can do whatever you want to.

The truth is that money cannot bring happiness, and certain people commit terrible acts because of their out of greed. It is essential to be part of all that. Don't be a snobby liar Do not make your life all about money. You have the power to decide how you're going to manage this money. Also, you have the ability to make sure that money doesn't dictate your life. And you must keep this in mind. Money can drive you to do crazy things, and we don't want you slide into that pit.

Mix the grind. Do your best to find an employment. I'm assuming you already have one. If not, you should get one. It is possible to set things up by yourself, but that is extremely difficult without a backup strategy. Therefore, try to set up one for a few days at the very least. If you can.

If you're employed that pays you, you've got money. Check with yourself to see if you're happy. If you're satisfied satisfied, you're free to skip this rule. If you'd like to make more money due to the fact that you are missing certain things in your life Start working on getting additional money as well.

It doesn't matter which way you go about it. Make sure you do it legally however, as you don't want in trouble. You can also trade stocks. If you want to learn about day trading. There are a myriad of possibilities. With your mindset and abilities. You are confident in yourself, you are confident that you can create something of it. Therefore, start.

Money allows you to be more independent. It offers more choices. You can even get fresh experiences. This ensures you don't need to stay in that job that you hate. Money is your greatest adversary, but it is important to approach it as an all-weather friend. There are so many different things that you can earn money from There are endless possibilities in reality. It's just a matter of finding the one that is right for you. You must find that one thing, that one area that you like so well that you can create something around it. You can then begin working again. Don't get too obsessed about it. If you want to earn passive income. I'll provide some suggestions and suggestions in the tips section.

Rule 25: Don't get distracted
It's easy to get caught up in the most insignificant things. YouTube videos and social media sites You know all. It's a complete unnecessary waste of time, and also mindless entertainment. It's okay to enjoy it at times. However, it's designed to be addicting. It's a long time to stay long, but what are you getting? You're losing time, and you get nothing.
This attitude is determined to be your best you and distractions don't belong there. The majority of mobile phones monitor the hours you're online per day. Check

that out and you'll likely be stunned, since you're unaware of how much time you're spending using your phone. You're just doing nothing but scrolling. You are allowed to unwind occasionally and browse Facebook and Twitter, it's completely normal. You shouldn't work continuously You'd be insane.

However, you must prioritize your work. It's not possible to be doing that thing all day long. You'll get more work done if take note of how often you're performing tasks that unnecessary.

I noticed it while writing this post I'm currently using YouTube and each time a song finishes, I go back to it and attempt to find a new one. It's possible to have a playlist to not be distracted, it's designed to be this way. It's time to free yourself from the hold it holds over you.

Rule 26: Quality over Quantity

If you consider through this thought process obviously you'd want high-quality over mass. The problem is that saying it's more straightforward than actually believing it.

When you concentrate on quality, your life will be more enjoyable. You can apply this principle to anything. Think of you are in the gym. I would rather you do 10 solid, solid repetitions instead of 12 quick ones. The quality of your work will help you improve. Quantity is just a numerical value.

Or, say friends. You could have 100 friends but do you actually have them? Are you seeking validation and only get it by having strange connections with a variety of people? It's obvious that having a few genuine friends is much more beneficial than having 100 friends you've known? You might believe that therefore why not apply the same principle to your life? Why limit yourself to Facebook or friends? Why not make your life more the best?

Quality also comes with the ability to be a deep. It's a lot. You will never to achieve if you concentrate exclusively on quantities. You can have everything but what exactly does it mean? Does it really be a thing?

That's the kind of question you have to ask yourself about the quality of.

The quality of life is, as I cannot be more clear the most effective choice. There are many things but you're working hard to obtain the best quality. Quantity is not the only thing that matters here. We are looking for the meaning, and you will only do that by focusing on high-quality.

The choice of quality can save you a ton of energy. The whole process is about reaching your objectives. It's hard enough on its own. Don't spend your time hunting unproductive shit, regardless of how tempting it might be. You're destroying your chances to win for nothing. If you focus on the highest quality, you'll receive high-quality. Think about it this way.

Quality is also linked to the principle of money. If you purchase only the things you require instead of purchasing useless crap then you save more money. This allows you to buy items to help you meet your goals. That's more valuable than the wooden spoon that you love.

The same goes for knowledge as well as your perception of things. You could go through 100 books, but honestly, how many of them will you keep in mind? What portion of the information is beneficial? It's a waste of time. We already have a shortage of time due to the fact that we work. Make sure you choose wisely. Pick the subjects you would like to grow in. If you want to relax, of course. But don't be tempted to read 100 book on the identical topic. Choose a high-quality one and make use of it to help you develop.

The pursuit of quality can make you healthier. Because you're always searching to find the top. Always searching for the top items and not stopping until you have them. The focus is on high-quality. It should be a pleasant experience and make you more efficient. In the end, you're better off seeking quality over quantity.

Rule 27, Don't be lost in the smallest pleasures
Small pleasures can be so addictive. Everybody has their personal items.

However, they can be distracting. The masturbation and gambling, social media and drinking. This is only draining you and robbing you of the potential. It doesn't bring you anything. Let me walk you through step-by-step the effects it has on you and why it's a bad idea.

Masturbation

It's not like that masturbating is harmful because it's actually good for you. The issue is the behaviour associated along with it. Sexualizing women is a bad idea which will make you feel fucked in the end since you'll begin to see women as goddesses. In fact, you might begin to think of them as nothing more than sexually attractive objects. It's not good. I'm not telling you to do it, but I'd even suggest you to do it, but not to do it constantly. Every once in a while perhaps? Be aware that the person you're cutting off is a human being too. Do not be a jerk Respect them the way you would yourself.

Social Media

I've already said it before, but look at all the fake life stories you see. It's all fake and can give you unrealistic expectations. People appear to think that their lives are perfect in the world, but it's not. They don't understand the struggles. They think that all is well and think that it's a way of life. However, don't get distracted by it and try not to get caught up in it. You could keep searching or you could be watching YouTube videos for hours on end, it's just a wasted time. Make sure to limit your time on YouTube or when you're relaxing. Don't let it control your life.

Gambling

It isn't clear if you have done this. Many people do it, but be aware. In the beginning, it could be extremely addictive. It all depends on how well you are at controlling yourself. However, it's also an unnecessary waste of time as with the rest. Sure, it's exciting to deposit a few dollars into a machine and then click buttons without thinking about it to experience the dopamine rush. This is because you're trying to achieve when gambling and winning. It's a great feeling however odds are not in your favor. This is designed to cause you to lose and, especially when you think about it this way it is best to be careful about it. It is a waste of time and potential when you do that, so put it aside and concentrate your energy for other things.

The alcohol itself does the talking for you. I'm not telling you to squander all the joy you have, but you shouldn't do that. However, you should be occupied with important shitman. If it's time to relax you can read an ebook or play games. Check out old pictures and talk to your grandparent You must keep up with that activity to stay in a good mood. Therefore, don't abandon that.

Do not get caught up in it. It's easy to forget the moment and forget that it's limited. The time is extremely valuable and, therefore, you should keep doing what you enjoy doing that you've always done and that were a joy to you. However, if you're trying to escape this kind of state, you have to be moving on, regardless of the situation. In other words, don't get caught up in the little pleasures. Keep looking at the larger perspective.

Rule 28 Fake it until achieve it.

Yep. This is against the entire ethos, however you must look more deeply into this.

If you don't believe in yourself then how do you expect to persevere? It's impossible. I don't care about whether you lie to yourself, you must in this scenario. It is possible that you don't believe in your self right now, but it's fine, right?

It's fine to doubt yourself, but it's important to put that doubt into the ground and then bury it. Because that doubt is likely hinder you and we can't afford the confidence to overcome it. You need to be sharp and have the motivation to continue. This isn't a valid reason when you don't believe in your abilities.

Learn to behave. Make yourself appear like the most confident momfucker on the block. You'll eventually be the person you want to become. That's why you rise up, that's why you work hard, and this is why you continue to work. Don't doubt you, even though do not. It's fine.

The process begins by affirming to yourself that you are the person you want to be. Even if that's a lie. Repeat it. You are exactly who you'd like to be. Again. The time is long enough to be able to believe that. Do you really care what other people think? Be honest about it. It is essential to believe in it in order for it to be effective. You will notice that once you have believed in for a long time you will actually become it. That's the method. You must trick your brain, and that will lead you to where you'd like to be.

Rule 29: Manage your emotions

It's not easy to control your emotions. If it wasn'tfor it, you wouldn't even be reading this garbage. Let me begin by saying that it's fine to be emotional. Human beings are human, and they can feel emotions. However, emotion can also be the reason you slip so deeply. It isn't a good idea to allow this to happen again on Therefore, you must to begin learning to manage this emotion. This includes emotions of all kinds like anger, sadness and all this shit. It needs to be controlled by you. You have to be the one who calls the shots and rather than the emotions. Be the one to take responsibility for your actions.

Then, take a look at the way that emotion affects your life. Note it down. You've lost relationships due to extreme emotions or just emotion generally, situations that you got caught up in because you weren't able to manage your emotions. Make a note of it and review it.

You must also learn to control your emotions. I'm guessing that you're stressed or depressed. It is possible that you have been suppressing your feelings for a while and aren't sure what to do no more. Be open about your feelings. You can even write each night prior to going to the bed, but you have to be able to acknowledge your feelings and acknowledge they exist.

After you have accept their existence, be patient until you feel extreme emotions. For instance, you become extremely angry for no apparent reason. You're tempted to wreck the entire house or breaking things. Don't. Take a moment to think.

Consider why you are feeling this in this way. What has caused you to become feel so terribly angry? It's possible that you're right. There's probably a valid reason to be mad. However do you really want allow it to control you? Are you planning to demolish your life because of it?

Find a better approach to deal with. At that point. If you're tempted to smash objects, or when you're ready to cry consider a better approach to deal with. For me I'm the gym guy. When I'm upset or sad, keep it in my locker and go to the gym. There's a way to deal with it too.

When you're in a position such as that, simply take a deep breath. Continue to practice it. Each time you feel extreme emotions, I'd like you to practice this shit. Simply breathe and think. Make use of that brain of yours. Know when to voice your emotions. Don't express your feelings when you're angry with someone and it will result in a sloppy argument that you'll need to resolve in the future. Not worth it. Allow yourself the time to relax. Whatever the difficulty is, I'm not worried. It is not possible to let emotions win. You must control it, and you can. If it requires you to get some time and be quiet, go for it. If you're looking to meditate and it improves your life then fuck it up. Simply be more mindful of your feelings and be able to manage it. That's all that is required.

Rule 30 Rule 30: Be the best person you can be.

The last rule of the mind and perhaps the most crucial one. All of those rules came to one point and that was to be the most perfect version of yourself. That's why I came up with the final rule. Everything revolved on this topic, all the time.

To be the most perfect self is vital. However, you must work towards it because it's not easy. Don't expect yourself to become the most perfect version of yourself right away. This process takes time, and I know that.

It is also necessary to start at the beginning and that's great too, as we all need to. There is a chance that you've suffered many times, everyone has their own tales. It's impossible to run an entire marathon without training so be patient with it. You're fine if the race isn't as fast as you'd hoped. Your vision is what matters. Not someone other people's. You're finally becoming yourself. Don't look for a secret trick or trick It's not there. It's up to you to make a difference in your life for yourself and only you. And I'm sure that, with these rules, you will be able to.

However, in the end I want you to develop into the greatest version of you. And I'm talking about the most perfect version you can be. Now and right today. You might feel down, but it's okay. You'll be able to get yourself up once more. Try to be the best that you can be right now, right? You can do it.

Chapter 8: Tip 1: Nobody Is Going To Be There To Help You.

Yes, it's painful does it not? The moment when you realize that you don't know what you're doing. The moment that all your best friends abandon you due to depression. It's not a good feeling, fist. However, it's something that you must learn to get stronger and be a solo wolf. In order to at least be able to carry it by yourself.

As I started my path, I hoped for at least one or two things to occur. It is either: A) My friends would be there and friendly as well) they would all gradually quit me and forget about me. If you chose B, you're right. Most left, as expected. My favorite friend stayed obviously; he is aware of the meaning of loyalty. The point is that you wish your friends would be there for you. If they do well, but I sure would like to think for them to do so. What kind of friend would leave other people in the dust? People who are weak-minded, honest.

Human nature is to avoid negative thoughts as quickly as is possible. They will come up with a variety of traits such as calling you toxic and so on. Whatever they can to escape the circumstance. You can't blame them But deep inside you are sure they are supposed to be there for you. But they're not.

It's a tough reality to accept, and it will hurt. I'm sure your family and friends are there and if they are, am so grateful for you. They are truly good people. But those who have left you today because you're down Remember them. Remember them when they ask for your assistance after you've developed to become the better version of yourself.

Because you'll come back more energized. They'll probably come back to tell you things like "I'm not able to remain in that negative environment and would you forgive me?', and then act like they didn't punch at you back. Man, I am going to be honest with you here however much you're missing them, don't allow people like them come back into your life. They didn't support your needs when they were most. Don't forget that they failed you. Just like I said that loyalty is an integral component of the sigma culture.

You've remained loyal to them for a few years. However, when the going got tough and they left, they walked away. There is no place for it in your mindset. It is crucial to be loyal.

However If you're just beginning this journey, then you're likely seeking help and support, and that is what you should. What I'm trying to convey is that you should do it by yourself. Many people claim they are willing to help but, in fact, they don't. It's just a method of making a formal statement, like"yes, I'll assist you. However, don't believe in me.

The assistance you get is fantastic However, do not rely on it as it will make you break up yet again. Only you are needed and nobody else will be able to take care of it. So, get rid of those who have left you, really. Also, be grateful to the ones who are standing by for you right now. Remember how they stood by your side when you were at your lowest.

Tip 2 Do not be afraid to take lessons from other people

This is something I wanted to clear. I'm sure that this attitude is centered on you and you alone. However, you shouldn't be put off taking lessons from other people. Everyone has their individual paths, and we each have our own paths and fates. Some people are farther along the way that we. They may not be exactly the same, but they've had to go through certain things.

They also dealt with the challenges. They developed their skills, interests and hobbies, whatever you want to call it. If you could save yourself by avoiding their errors, then why should you not try it? People can be a great teacher. Particularly, elderly people. They've been through the world. They know what has to be done in order to get the job done. They got old because of reasons. It could be that it's because they were with an accomplice and life was simpler back then however it wasn't. All of us have difficulties, we all face challenges and demons of our own.

They worked hard they required to find a suitable partner. Of course, there were some who had more success than others. However, not every advice will be the best advice you've have ever received. However, taking it into account isn't going to harm you. The most likely thing to be the case is that you aren't happy with the idea, however it could provide valuable information.

You can also transmit the information. In the guidelines Knowledge is power. It makes you appear more attractive. The more you are aware the more you know, the more you know. You could be an inspiration to someone somewhere else in the future.

Tip 3. Your opinion is important.
We are not talking about some crappy survey here. It's about me and what you've got to say. It doesn't matter

regardless of what other people say to you.

It's not hard to believe that it's best to not talk when others are discussing. If you are asked to share your thoughts you'll agree with what you heard from someone who is not you. It's easier, and they will not be able to make fun of your thoughts.

You must quit thinking that way and start believing that your opinions do really matter. It doesn't matter whether you believe it's foolish, or when they say it's stupid and it's not even going to matter what anyone else believes. If the entire world believes that your view is nonsense, don't bother. It is important to believe in the value of your opinion. It is your responsibility to prove to the world that you have faith in your ideals.

This is also a an aspect of confidence. Man doesn't bow to and follow the dictates of other people. No. Do not be a follower. become an authority. A leader's opinion is expressed with complete confidence. Every word that is spoken from the mouth of a leader has been considered. I want you to do the same.

It's all an idea. If you'd prefer to remain still, it's fine. Be aware that your opinion is important and you're free to express your opinion, even if other people aren't keen to listen to what you say. It's up to you.

Tip 4: Don't overwork yourself
It's not even speaking about the mind-set. I'm talking about the general issue this article. Because it's easy to work too much yourself. We're expected to be on the job all day and be relentless regardless of what.

And with this suggestion I'm sure it's against the general mindset. But I'm going to have to incorporate it into. If you don't keep an eye on it and actually work yourself too hard then you'll end up being in a bind. You'll be exhausted and depressed once more, so please be cautious.

No matter how many tasks you need to accomplish or the number of goals you've set By overworking yourself, you're not doing harm to anyone. You're only hurting yourself. Stay focused on your goals and recognize that you won't be able to accomplish your goals if you're stressed out and overworked in the long term. Always think in the long term.

Also, of course, offer everything you've got. You should push yourself to the absolute limit, and the rest. The limit is just that, the limit, and it should be treated in the same way as the limits. Don't exceed it, unless you have the need to. The future you may require the energy therefore don't take it away from it.

The habits you build today are the ones you'll take with you to the next. If you are a night-crawler to finish your work How are you going to be able to accomplish that next time around? It's likely to be the same. Start by developing the right habits for your work today to ensure that the future will be able to gain from it. Get yourself set for success.

Tip 5: Workout!

This is one of my top tips and I can't wait to share it with you. I enjoy exercising and working out at the gym. If you've never gone to the gym it is difficult to get started. Therefore, I will explain what it is that the gym is all about and how it operates and what's the best option for beginners, and all that.

In the beginning, what you should exercise in contrast to the norm?

The gym is a great resource to aid you in losing weight. If you are looking to shed fat or to build muscle it is possible to do both in the fitness center. It's all in the amount of effort you put into it! Diet is a key factor in this, and we'll talk about it in the following article, but they do work hand-in-hand. There is no way to gain or lose weight by not hitting the exercise routine.

Being fit can help in fighting off diseases and health problems. Your body is stronger than average due to the exercise. It's not just about physical health! Exercise is also a great way to combat anxiety and depression. You need to have a solid foundation to build a fresh you. So this can be a fantastic start!

The gym can also be an ideal place to let off some steam. In order to get the anger and anger out of your system and feel less anxious exercising produces positive chemical changes in your brain which help you feel more relaxed. This isn't a magical solution getting to the gym for a few minutes won't fix your anxiety, yet if stick to it as a part of your routine, it will be beneficial.

Training for a workout can also help to boost your level of energy! It can make you feel tired, and it can, however it also an energy booster. This is a long-term thing but. Your body is getting stronger, so you can do your everyday tasks also. It might not be evident immediately however, you will notice it within a couple of months. Things will become much more simple and go more smoothly. You are free from too much stress, and, yes, it does boost your energy levels. Stress is tiring. I'd rather channel that energy into my gym to feel better , instead of being exhausted. A more robust heart and healthier lung capacity will help you get moving and make getting up much easier and it's win-win! A lower stress level and more positive energy.

It is also very helpful with sleeping. I don't know about you but I have a hard time trying to sleep. I'm always overwhelmed by things in my life, and all other stuff.. This keeps me awake at late at night. However, when I exercise and are able to let go of tension at fitness, I fall asleep well. I'm exhausted however, I also shed some of the stress that comes with it. This has helped me sleep better and that's great in your mood, too.

I'm not sure whether you have a spouse currently. There will be one in the near future however. It's not a good idea to look sloppy in sex, and you'll look more attractive when you workout. Everything is in place and makes it worthwhile. Your odds of getting erectile dysfunction will be lower when you exercise.

And lastly, the enjoyment you get from working out! It might feel like a chore in the beginning however once you begin realizing the results, you'll enjoy going to the fitness center. It's also fun particularly if you go to the gym regularly! You can also meet new people and chat with others and it's great for your social life as well!

The most important thing to remember is that exercise is good for both your mental and physical well-being. That's enough reason to begin going to the fitness center even if it's just once or twice every week. Every single thing you do is important.

I hope that this gave the motivation you needed to get moving. We must first to look at the goals you'd like to reach.

Are you looking to build strength? To increase size? For strength and strength? Are you looking to shed the weight or increase it? Do you wish to appear healthy? The first chapter will focus on size and strength. The gain or lose weight discussion will occur within the following chapter.

In simple terms it is all about the production of force. Size however is about creating an energy pump that causes tiny injuries to the muscle that is then causing it to repair and get bigger. This is the definition of hypertrophy.' (1)

Keep in mind that when you train to build size, you will naturally become stronger as well. They are both connected however they operate in different ways. It's all about what you'd like to be. Do you wish to be large and powerful or just strong?

The general principle to follow when training to build strength is that the reps should be small and the load of resistance must be heavy. Additionally, true low-rep strength training is mostly neuromuscular. If you consider the body's computer, then strength exercises are more concerned with improving your software that is part of your central nervous system (CNS) rather than it is about the hardware, your muscles. Training for strength is about instructing the CNS how to add more muscles into the game or to boost motor unit activation.' (1)

I hope this makes sense to you today. Personally, I prefer to train to build strength and size. I am awestruck by how my body appears when I workout and it makes sense to follow that path If you're looking to embrace the principles completely. It's all about making the most of yourself, and I'm assuming you're looking to see the improvements. However, if you simply want to improve your strengths, that's cool too!

"Bodybuilding isn't about becoming an "weightlifter." The focus is on using the weights to build muscle. By putting as much weight on the bar as you can, whether to boost your confidence or impress your friends is not the right device to accomplish the task.' (1)

This is basically what the mentality is trying to teach you. Be aware of these things and remain there for you as well as your height. It is important to remember that you must challenge yourself but not in a manner that makes you appear like a sexy jerk trying to impress people.

The last thing I'd like to demonstrate before you're ready for your journey

When you're way too much, here's what happens:

* You decrease the amount of duration of tension because you're forced to utilize the momentum of your opponent to win.
* You're not able to reduce your weight with a steady and controlled manner which will further reduce your time in tension.
* You're not able to concentrate on the muscles that are being worked due to the fact that you struggle just to lift that weight on.
* You use additional muscles. It decreases the amount of muscle pump you want to concentrate on.' (1)

There was quite a bit of talk and it's not a bad thing. If you're looking to go to the gym as well as possible, you must to be aware of these things before you mess up your back or appear like clowns.

Then, you're likely to begin with the gym. There are 3 basic exercises that are the gold cows in the gym: The bench press that hits your chest muscles, deadlift that targets the back muscles and the squat which targets the leg muscles.

These compound exercises work several other muscles. For instance, when you bench press, you will also strengthen your triceps. Squatting can help strengthen the abs, your core and the list goes on. Three of them are important exercises, and you'll soon be being asked a lot about your bench. Do not get caught up in the exercise, master your techniques first. Check out YouTube videos on the proper method. The most important aspect, poor technique can cause you to be a mess in the end and we don't want that.

Personally, I am a huge believer that I am a huge believer in PPL (Push the Legs) program. I do this at least twice every week, and go to the gym six times per week.

The push is focused on chest shoulders, triceps, and chest. The majority of exercises are linked. The pull is directed at your biceps. Back and legs are directed at your legs.

(2)

This is a program that you could try to start your journey. My method is slightly different, however I've been working out for a long time , so I'm naturally much heavier. Don't be fooled by the fact that this program isn't tough! I've added it because I think this program to be a great choice. If you are not happy then you can search for a different program via Google.

A few suggestions I could provide are: you will be able to see some exercises, but you'll have no clue on how to perform them. That's fine. A similar exercise to that of the Romanian deadlift that I haven't done. The good thing is that the internet is brimming with alternatives. There are a lot of exercises, and you could search for an exercise that is less complicated and targets those same muscle groups. I was there too, I do it every occasionally. You go into the fitness center to let off the stress, not worry about your workouts.

The final and most important tip. When you fill out your registration make sure to inquire whether the staff can provide support. Your application is so importantthat it can hurt you or cause damage more vulnerable in the end. If there's no one to assist you, get someone else to examine. If you're hesitant to do this, look up on YouTube the best way to exercise. be carried out.

Tip 6: Nutrition

The nutrition component is around 50 percent of your training. Growth is created in the kitchen and in the exercise room. One cannot go without the other, so let's take a the time to look over the things you should know about.

The first thing to note is that there are three types of diet plans. It is possible to bulk, which means you gain weight in the form of muscles. The fat gain is not significant, however, you'll gain someweight, and there's no stopping it. It's not a issue. It will allow you to increase in size and increase muscles mass.

Weight maintenance is as simple as it. You eat, you remain at the same size, however you'll gain strength. I generally do this on days off since you're not burning many calories and there's no need to bulk or cutting. If you'd like to get serious, you can do that on even on rest days, but I'm not going to stress about it during those times.

Cutting is eating fewer calories than you consume. This can make you lose weight and appear more toned, but if you screw this up , you could also lose muscle. Be careful about it.

There is no universal definition of what is bulking and cutting. Bulking is having more food than you'll need to gain pounds, and then build muscle by doing resistance exercise. Cutting is eating less fat than the calories you consume (and likely exercising more) so that you can shed the fat. The idea behind it is that you build more muscle and fat and then shed the fat, making you appear slim and toned.' (3)

To increase the size of your muscles in order to build muscle mass, you need to "eat greater calories that are you need to maintain your weight" says your personal fitness coach Scott Laidler. "A significant portion of your calories come from food that contains protein that will provide you with the amino acids needed to increase muscles mass. If you don't have protein, you'll simply gain fat and gain less muscles" He continues. However, there is some limit.

It's not as easy since muscle equals protein. "There exists a genetic limit in the amount of muscle mass you are able to build at a particular period of time, regardless of how vigorously you workout and consume protein" according to the weight loss coach and personal trainer Dr. Aishah Muhammad. Therefore, if you eat too much, you'll gain weight.' (3)

It's pretty difficult to shed all the fat you'd like while maintaining muscles when cutting.

A few years ago, scientists discovered that one weight of fat is 3500 pounds of calories. However, burning just one pounds of your fat body mass isn't so easy as cutting down your calories by that much Your body is a lover of make muscle. Scott Laidler learned this from his own experience as he began his journey in the fitness field. He explained, "When I cut I did not consume enough calories and consequently took off some from the mass I gained. The phases would cross paths for a couple of weeks, in which I would look and feel great, however I wanted to be slim and strong all the time. It wasn't a great experience." (3)

You now are aware of what it all is and how it functions in large lines.

When you begin your diet, you have to ensure that you monitor your macros. You can go all-out and keep track of every calorie. That's the way I go. You can download an app for food on the Google Play Store to track your calories.

I hear a lot of people claim that they are eating enough, yet they aren't gaining the weight they want, and how could that possible. The answer is simple, you aren't eating enough. Even if you think you're eating more than you should various factors influence the ways you lose or gain muscles. Metabolism, weight now, length etc.

First, you need to determine how many calories you require each day. This can be done by searching for a calculator using Google. I personally prefer this one because it's very simple:

'https://www.calculator.net/calorie-calculator.html'

Simply enter your body weight, height, and activity level , and boom it calculates everything for you. It's as simple as that. Be aware that you must keep track of your calories consumption.

It's not easy, and, believe me when I say that it can get boring. However, if you're willing to do everything you can for this, it's the best choice. If you prefer to relax and prefer to workout to enjoy the pleasure of exercising it's fine too. You just need to eat some more. Don't forget to eat plenty of protein! Google offers a ton of information that I'm not able to give you however, these top three ones.

Tip 7: Make sure you keep your home spotless

This may sound like a small thing that's not, but it really can make a huge impact. If you're anything like me, you throw all your trash onto the floor. You heap up the dishes, and you throw your clothes all over the place and then you're not sure where. It's a common occurrence we all have.

Trust me when I say that it is a pleasure when you arrive home to a tidy house. Instead of having to deal by a huge mess and stressing yourself out it is possible to relax and relax and do what you love without worrying.

It's also much healthier for you. The dust that's in the air really stinks. Insects are attracted by it.. It's not a good idea to have this kind of shit to be in your house. There is no need to do that.

Think about when you invite someone over. When you finally meet the person who truly means everything to you, you'll need to be stressed or cancel the date because you are unable to be in time. It's a huge hassle would it not?

It also eliminates the hassle of constantly looking for your belongings. From personal experience, I can tell you that I'm spending around 15 minutes a day looking for items. Where was my coat, what is my keys, etc. I'm already stressed enough therefore it's a waste of time to be stressed out yet again.

Make it part of your daily routine. Your home represents you If your home is messy as is your lifestyle. Make sure you clean it up and place things back where they belong.

Tip 8. Negativity is an option.

It might appear to be a different thing however it is. It's your choice what you think about things and how you handle them.

Yes, things are bound to turn bad. There's no way to prevent this from happening. Bad things is bound to happen to you and it happens to everybody. But , you have to remember that everyone has their own method to handle it. You could be acting in a unhealthy manner.

You can learn how to feel more confident in your outlook on the world around you.

Every issue is not an issue. There is a lot to gain from problems. It all depends on how you handle it. If you are looking at it from a negative perspective or with the thought that it could be an opportunity to create something new?

Look for the positive aspects of a negative situation. Negative points will be an overhand. That's the reason it's a negative situation, however there is plenty of positives. Focus on the positive aspects first. When you can see the good in them take a moment to be thankful for them. Recognize the fact that they exist. The situation that is bad will pass eventually and the good ones can remain if you treat them in a positive way. Do not put everything in one corner.

The majority of situations are really bad. You hate them. However, you must admit that some are amusing. Consider all of the factors you had to go wrong to get into this situation. It seems like a silly joke. Try to think of it in this way. This isn't the end of the world.

Tip 9 Tip 9: Passive income

It's always a good idea to have some cash and some sort of income. The most efficient method of earning money is to have a passive income, which is money that which you don't have to earn, but instead by an arrangement you make for the long-term.

I'll provide you with a few suggestions. This isn't financial advice, by any means and you must be aware that everything has risk. It is possible to lose everything quickly with just a few suggestions other ideas are better but take longer. It's all in what you're trying to accomplish.

You can begin by selling something that you make as a hobby. For instance, this book for example. While I'm not doing it to earn cash, and that's the reason why I set it at a low price however, it does serve some purpose and also makes me money even when I'm sleeping or out of the house. It's an asset that earns cash. The difference between books and other assets is since the amount is determined by the amount of people who purchase instead of how many they are. They are printed at any point. However, you can create courses or any other document that you could offer to customers. The idea is to create assets, however the risk remains. But, if it's something you really love, it's an excellent idea.

Another option is the rental income. However, I doubt anyone of you has the money to buy houses, so let's skip the rental income. Be aware that it's an option to consider in the event that you have enough money to purchase an additional house and rent it out.

Another option is affiliate marketing. You sell products of other people and earn an amount of money for it. There are a lot of sites that permit you to join as an affiliate, but you need to decide whether you'd like to be an individual's Pawn. If you have an extensive Instagram account, or any other type of account you have, you could always add your affiliate link in your bio to see what you can earn. This isn't my kind of passive income , but should it be a good fit for you do it!

Another option is to invest in crypto or stocks. I would recommend being very cautious with crypto because it is basically gambling. Bitcoin appears to be an investment that is relatively safe, but it could end soon too. Stocks are certainly the safest choice and your portfolio could be growing by as much as 5 percent annually. It's not much , but it's better as opposed to the rental the bank pays you. The bank is risk-free but that's the cost you pay. If you choose to put your money into stocks like Google and Apple I'm sure you'll be perfectly safe. However, I would strongly suggest you to investigate the stocks you're planning decide to put your money into. Don't trust me to tell you what I think.

If you're a programmer and this is your pastime then you could make an app that is simple. It's free, you can put advertisements on it, and watch the money roll in. It takes a lot of effort to create something amazing, but, if it's your passion is it really that important? If you enjoyed it, then great! If it fails it was fun, and that's all that matters.

Tip 10: A sport can be life-saving.
It's not regarding fitness. But that is also great. But I'm talking about a football team or whatever sport you prefer.
I'm personally a huge football fan. It is extremely intense and a large amount of emotion goes along in it. And , you know what is the best part? It helps me to sleep. It makes me sleep better during the day because I know that I will quickly watch my team play again. It's another reason to rise and continue to work. Since the team has stood by me even if they didn't know me, they'd be disappointed in my help. Why should I abandon my cause? If they were in a slump they fought to climb back on their feet. Why why don't you fight?
It also can increase your connection with your fellow players. In Europe there are a lot of people who love football. There is always discuss it and it isn't a matter of

who you are as long as you're supporting the same club, it's family.

It's all about uniting. When you put on your shirt and step into the crowd of crows wearing the shirt you'll feel like a godsend. Everyone in the vicinity has your back and you do not even know who they are.

In the world of sports there is no distinction between the person you are or where you're from. All it boils down to sharing the same goal and that's what unites you. As odd as it sounds you should give it a go. If you go to the stadium or visit an establishment during the game you'll be able to meet many new people who will appreciate your attire and colors. This is the easiest method to connect with people.

Tip 11: Professional assistance is fine
I am sure you're thinking. It's not true If you're like me, you're averse to professional assistance. You're trying to resolve your own issues and you don't

want to burden others , and you're not interested in medication or talking to someone. This is just dumb and taking a pill to get better. What's do you think? This isn't human.

Now, I'm not sure. When I was first thinking about it, I thought this too. The whole thing about the mind could help get you free of depression. But it's not guaranteed to do so. If it doesn't happen mean that you're already away. It's fine. It happened to you and me too It happened to everyone.

These people are eager to assist you. They will. They can assist you in dealing with issues that arise in your life. They can help you feel stronger Some are so great, they could help you to find your life's goals. Whatever you'd like to accomplish, they will take it away from you. And I did my best. This method worked for me However, if it isn't working help you, you should seek professional assistance. There's nothing wrong with this. Being honest enough to admit you're struggling is an extremely significant and bold step. And there are times when we aren't able to solve problems by ourselves. Therefore, why not take the help of professionals who are paid? You see, they are money for their services, which is why they are eager to assist you. It's part of their job.

The majority of people who seek treatment find themselves feeling better. As an example, over 80 percent of patients who receive treatment for depression recover. The treatment for anxiety disorders can have up to 90 percent chance of success. It's certainly worthwhile to try.

Tip 12: Do not self-medicate
Self-medicating is the process of managing personal problems like emotional pain, depression or even sadness with the help of drugs, medications or alcohol.

It can be tempting, definitely. When I am feeling down, I'm also tempted to take some painkillers, or even drink alcohol. But , it's not possible to do this. Since after a time it becomes an habit. You're now in dangerous territory when you reach this point. It is not a good idea to get addicted to something.

Alcohol is your sole substance that can ease your pain, sure, you're likely to drink more alcohol. Then, eventually, the substance will get into a spiral that is out of control, and you'll be hooked or be faced with health problems. It's absolutely not worth it even if it dulls you right now. This is the short-term solution. In the long run, you'll have to deal with a lot more issues due to this. So seriously, avoid it.

Find ways to be healthy and cope with your current feelings no matter how challenging it might be. I feel the same way I truly do. I tried it for a few months in the alcohol world as well. However, it only caused me to get sicker, and eventually I was forced to end it up as well. At the end of the day I managed to numb my pain for short time however, I did not gain anything beneficial from the experience. My issues only grew.

It's not something I want to occur to you. As I mentioned look for more healthy ways to live. Develop that feeling and keep it for your fitness center. Try meditation I don't even know. Don't make yourself a mess with things like this.

Tip 13 Tip 13: Learn a new language
If you already know one, fantastic! Take another course. This is also a way of focusing on enhancing your abilities and learning more, and it is certainly one of the ways!

Learning more than one language could greatly benefit your career. It can make you worth much more. I've stated it before, knowing is power, and this is certainly true for learning a new language. It's also beneficial for brain's function!

There are numerous online tools to help you learn a language, including Duolingo. I wouldn't recommend it as many courses only give you a few random words and then you do nothing but the same thing.

There are a lot of YouTube videos to begin to learn. It is important to learn the pronunciation of every letter and understand how grammar functions. Once you understand this, it's a lot simpler. When you are able to understand the structure of sentences and how sentences are constructed, you can test your reading skills in the language you're trying to master. This could be a good exam for yourself!

In terms of which language to learn you should check out the most widely spoken languages around the globe. I would strongly suggest Spanish as it's a language widely spoken in many countries. It's also easy to master even if you already know English.

If you're looking for a true test, you should try Russian! When you've learned it, it's an amazing language. However, due to their alphabet, their accents and the alphabet, it's difficult to master. It can put you up to a serious challenging task, and if that's the goal you are after, why not?

Tip 14: Don't make assumptions about others.

Human nature is to categorize people. It's simpler to understand and explain their actions. Yes, he does act as he does because of this or this. No. It's time to put an end to this. What are your feelings when someone criticizes you? Based on the look of your actions?

You can say that you are depressed. This is what they call you as depressed and fucking savage. They don't see the potential of you and your abilities. They deliberately ignore it because it's unclear to them. They must place a label on you in order to comprehend your personality. I'm guessing you don't like this, and it's time to put it down in a serious manner. It's just not fair.

There's a theory that claims that you act according to the label you are given. If people continually criticize you for being dumb, you will eventually appear dumb. Since we are conditioned to adhere to the stereotypes we are given. I'm not sure what the reason is, but, hey, science. Labels are basically all-or-nothing. If you believe that people can alter, you will be less self-conscious about your own self. You may not be aware of that you have labeled yourself as well.

The idea is to take the time to look at people for what they are. If someone says something that isn't true isn't a sign that they're stupid. Don't think about them as the way they are. Look at everything they can offer and assess each step in a different way. You'd want this for yourself So, do it to other people as well. The world will appear different when you see people in this way. It opens an ocean of possibilities and possibilities.

Tip 15: Read books.

It doesn't matter which book you choose to read is crucial. It assists in developing more vocabulary, and it improves your thinking ability and assists in focusing. It can also help you become more empathic from reading books! There are plenty of other mental advantages that we cannot all talk about and you'll have to trust me or look them up.

It is recommended to read every day for at minimum thirty minutes each day. You'll surely reap benefits. Make sure to read before going to bed, and it's beneficial to end your day with a great book since it is usually quite well.

It's the same as what I said to you to think about. The most successful people have a habit of reading books. I'm not sure why, but reading books does not guarantee you the next Bill Gates or anything, but there's so much information in books. Also, try reading books written by people who motivate you, who have had walked the path you would like to take, people who share the same values. It can get you excited and you'll want that. Books, specifically non-fiction can give the best advice in the realm of the world of. You will need it when you're on the road.

If you spend 30 minutes reading each day, you can take up to 50 books in a year. This is a huge amount of knowledge. And who knows what you'll benefit from it. Particularly when you read works written by or about people who will inspire you. You'll be a speedy reader in time and there are many advantages to this.

Tip 16: Get 8-10 hours per night.

It's easy to fall off the sleep. Reduce it to 6 or 7 hours per night. This isn't enough, and eventually it's going to make you break. When you're working out and you'll need more hours than. Ideally, 10. But 8 , for you if it's the highest you can fit in. It is important to get back into shape after the weights and heavy lifting regardless of whether you're lifting your emotions or weights. It's just that you really need to take a break.

It's also vital to our immune system. This shit weakens as time passes because it's doing its job at a high rate. If you're doing that you'll get exhausted as well. Also, make sure that your body gets relaxation too.

It's not just your body, though. Your head needs energy, too. If you don't have energy, it's difficult to concentrate. Consider the time you fell asleep really poor and how much difficulty it was to concentrate the next day after. Take a look at what you could gain from having a regular and healthy sleeping schedule. It is possible that you are running through the air and your body has been adjusting to it however, what's the purpose? You're looking to perform at the highest level, right? That's why you require that vitality, that concentration. It's all about sleep.

And one more important point. Sleep helps against depression. Set yourself up on a regular schedule and don't fail yourself. Do your best to sleep 8-10 hours a night and you'll see over time, your life will be transformed. If it doesn't, then what do you stand to lose? Perhaps a couple of hours?

Tip 17: Don't overdo it.

The mind is an excellent way to overcome depression. And I know you'd like to take advantage of it as soon as you can. You wish to be feeling better as soon as you can and that's perfectly normal. However, I'd like to share with you an incident that occurred to me a few years ago due to me going too far with my mentality.

This is why the mind tells us to go on regardless of what. In a way, that might be the right decision to make. However, I was way too out of my comfort zone with it. I was experiencing terrible pain. My back hurt so badly that I had to wake up numerous times because of the discomfort. It was a nightmare and I couldn't walk due to it hurting so much.

In addition I also had an illness. The first thing to note is that this was really up.

Secondly, it made me feel even worse. I couldn't breathe through my nose , and yes, I was sick and wanted to stay in bed. The feeling was not right.

Therefore, I chose to go at home the next day. At first. I was sitting in my room I was contemplating writing but was not feeling it. I was forced to take action or do something. I didn't know which was the best approach to take.

I decided later to take a shower to try to see if it would aid, or even help generally. I got in the shower and felt fine. It wasn't perfect, but it was a little better at the very least.

However, I could not remain silent and sit around throughout the day. I needed to leave. So I searched my wardrobe, searching for any medicine. Painkillers, uppers, whatever I could discover. I found aspirin as well as some pre-workout. I decided to mix them together. It eased my discomfort for a while however it wasn't nearly enough. I still felt horrible.

www.ingramcontent.com/pod-product-compliance
Lightning Source LLC
Chambersburg PA
CBHW050024130526
44590CB00042B/1895